The Wounded Storyteller

ARTHUR W. FRANK

The Wounded Storyteller

BODY,
ILLNESS,
AND
ETHICS

THE UNIVERSITY
OF CHICAGO PRESS
CHICAGO AND LONDON

Arthur Frank is the author of *At the Will of Body: Reflections on Illness*. He lives in Calgary, Alberta, where he teaches sociology at the University of Calgary.

The University of Chicago Press, Chicago 60637
The University of Chicago Press, Ltd., London
© 1995 by The University of Chicago
All rights reserved. Published 1995
Printed in the United States of America
04 03 02 01 00 99 98 97 96 95   1 2 3 4 5

ISBN (cloth) 0-226-25992-7

Library of Congress Cataloging-in-Publication Data

Frank, Arthur W.
   The wounded storyteller : body, illness, and ethics / Arthur W. Frank.
      p.   cm.
   Includes index.
   ISBN 0-226-25992-7
   1. Sick—Psychology.   2. Discourse analysis, Narrative.
   I. Title.
   R726.5.F726   1995
   306.4′61—dc20   95–12989
                                                              CIP

♾ The paper used in this publication meets the
minimum requirements of the American National Standard
for Information Sciences—Permanence of Paper for
Printed Library Materials, ANSI Z39.48–1984.

To my parents,
Jane and Arthur Frank,
in their fifty-fourth year of marriage.

*All they had was mine,
and they are with me always.*

. . . I had grasped well that there are situations in life where our body is our entire self and our fate. I was in my body and nothing else. . . . My body . . . was my calamity. My body . . . was my physical and metaphysical dignity.

Jean Améry[1]

Contents

Preface

The figure of the wounded storyteller is ancient: Tiresias, the seer who reveals to Oedipus the true story of whose son he is, has been blinded by the gods. His wound gives him his narrative power. The wound that the biblical patriarch Jacob suffers to his hip while wrestling with the angel is part of the story he tells of that event, and it is the price of his story. As Jacob tells his story to those he returns to—and who else could have told it?—his wound is evidence of his story's truth.

This book presents ill people as wounded storytellers. I hope to shift the dominant cultural conception of illness away from passivity—the ill person as "victim of" disease and then recipient of care—toward activity. The ill person who turns illness into story transforms fate into experience; the disease that sets the body apart from others becomes, in the story, the common bond of suffering that joins bodies in their shared vulnerability.

The emphasis of contemporary writing is less on the wounded storyteller than on the complementary figure of the wounded healer. For example, Henri Nouwen's *The Wounded Healer* bases the spiritual vocation on the minister's acceptance and sharing of her own woundedness.[1] Physicians from Arthur Kleinman to Larry Dossey and journalists like Bill Moyers present the wounded healer as an ideal for medical workers.[2] Rita Charon writes of the physician's need "to allow our own injuries to increase the potency of our care of patients, to allow our personal experiences to strengthen the empathic bond with others who suffer."[3]

Charon can be read equally well as describing the ill person's need. As wounded, people may be cared for, but as story-tellers, they care for others. The ill, and all those who suffer, can also be healers. Their injuries become the source of the potency of their stories. Through their stories, the ill create empathic bonds between themselves and their listeners. These bonds expand as the stories are retold. Those who listened then tell others, and the circle of shared experience widens. Because stories can heal, the wounded healer and wounded storyteller are not separate, but are different aspects of the same figure.

But telling does not come easy, and neither does listening. Seriously ill people are wounded not just in body but in voice. They need to become storytellers in order to recover the voices that illness and its treatment often take away. The voice speaks the mind and expresses the spirit, but it is also a physical organ of the body. The mystery of illness stories is their expression of the body: in the silences between words, the tissues speak. This book is about hearing the body in the ill person's speech.

The chapters below begin with how illness requires stories, the body as the ground of these stories, and illness stories as what are called self-stories. The middle chapters describe three narrative types of illness stories, understanding these narratives as ways of using the body. These middle chapters suggest what illness stories tell; the final chapters move to the force of that telling. They locate the ethical imperative of illness stories in issues of testimony and witness.

In wounded storytelling the physical act becomes the ethical act. Kierkegaard wrote of the ethical person as editor of his life: to tell one's life is to assume responsibility for that life.[4] This responsibility expands. In stories, the teller not only recovers her voice; she becomes a witness to the conditions that rob others of their voices. When any person recovers his voice, many people begin to speak through that story.

Stories of people trying to sort out who they are figure prominently on the landscape of postmodern times. Those who have been objects of others' reports are now telling their own stories. As they do so, they define the ethic of our times: an ethic of voice, affording each a right to speak her own truth, in her own words.

This book is a work of theory, but it is equally a collection of stories and a kind of memoir. For almost a decade I have been a wounded storyteller, and I have cultivated the stories of others who are wounded, each in different ways. The "theory" in this book elaborates my story and theirs.

Charles Lemert introduces his social theory textbook by calling theory "a basic survival skill."[5] *The Wounded Storyteller* is a survival kit, put together out of my need to make sense of my own survival, as I watch others seeking to make sense of theirs. The wounded storyteller, like Lemert's theorist, is trying to survive and help others survive in a world that does not immediately make sense.

Sooner or later, everyone is a wounded storyteller. In postmodern times that identity is our promise and responsibility, our calamity and dignity. The "theory" I propose here is one tool kit to help fulfill that promise and exercise that responsibility. Twenty years ago when I was a graduate student, theories were proposed with the tag line that they awaited "further research." I now prefer the idea that this theory awaits further living and the stories of those lives. The theory has been shaped by the stories I have been privileged to live and to hear, and I encourage readers to reshape it in the same spirit.

Acknowledgments

Any book is written out of many relationships, and this one has particularly personal debts.

My first thanks go to all the people who have told me their stories of illness. I hope this book honors not just those stories I have been able to quote, but also the many others that taught me what I know about illness.

At Calgary, my friend and head of department, Richard Wanner, has shared this project personally and supported it professionally. Lynda Costello's cheerfulness has been as valuable as her logistical help.

This book was developed in presentations given in response to more invitations than I can acknowledge here. For their particular opportunities and generosity, I thank Dr. Andrew Achenbaum, Institute of Gerontology, University of Michigan; Dr. Ruth Buczynski, National Institute for the Clinical Application of Behavioral Medicine; Dr. Larry Burton and JoAnn O'Reilly, Rush University and Rush-Presbyterian-St. Luke's Medical Center, Chicago; Judy Gerner, Director, The Anderson Network, M. D. Anderson Cancer Center, Houston; Dr. Ross Gray, The Toronto-Bayview Regional Cancer Centre; Dr. Sue Marsden, Hospice New Zealand; Dr. Balfour Mount, International Congress for the Care of the Terminally Ill, Montreal; and Harold Robles, Director, The Albert Schweitzer Institute for the Humanities, Hamden, Connecticut.

Academic colleagues have offered not just scholarly opinions, but in many cases have added their own stories to support those I have presented. I thank people not only for their collegiality but for their fellowship. Although no material is reprinted from my earlier writings, many ideas presented here were first developed in journal articles written with the kind encouragement of the editors. Thanks to Norman Denzin, as editor of both *Studies in Symbolic Interaction* and *The Sociological Quarterly;* Kathryn Montgomery Hunter, *Literature and Medicine;* and Hank Stam, *Theory & Psychology.* My writing on the body began at the invitation of Mike Featherstone, *Theory, Culture & Society,* and would not have been possible without the earlier work of Bryan Turner, who is among the most undercited influences on this book.

My editors and good friends at *Second Opinion: Health, Faith, Ethics,* are Barbara Hofmaier, Sandy Pittman, and Martin Marty, senior editor. They have shaped my thinking and my writing through their editing of my own essays, in review projects, and in our joint editing of the "Case Stories" series. Thanks also to Ron Hamel and Edwin DuBose. My extensive debts to Martin Marty include the writing I have done for *The Christian Century,* where he and David Heim have sent me excellent books for review.

Good books have also arrived regularly from another friend, John Hofsess, editor of *Last Rights,* Victoria, British Columbia, and several of these are cited below.

The earliest draft of this book received extensive comments from Anne Hunsaker Hawkins, Susan DiGiacomo, and from my father, Arthur W. Frank, Jr. As I write below, few scholars have contributed as much to the public hearing of illness stories as Anne has. Susan read my work both as a social scientist and as a person who has had cancer. I thank her for the commitment we share to the interdependence of those roles. My father reminded me what a non-academic reader would see in my "perfectly clear" text. He and Susan helped me remember who the book was written for.

Readers of later drafts included Robert Zussman and Arthur Kleinman. Robert's reading was the beginning of a friendship, while Arthur's was another culmination in a relationship that has pushed me in new directions during the last five years. As numerous as citations to Arthur's work are in this book, they only begin to express his influence on my writing. I emphasize that all these readers saw and commented on drafts; to adapt one of my favorite phrases of Robert Zussman's, their liability for the final version should be limited.

The final draft of the book was guided by Richard Allen, acting as manuscript editor. Richard's sensitivity to what my prose was attempting, his own expertise about narrative and ethics, and our shared commitment to accessibility in intellectual writing led to a most gratifying collaboration.

My editor at Chicago was Douglas Mitchell, with whom I have enjoyed sharing ideas about books for the last decade. Beyond his breadth of knowledge and wit, Doug gives an author the best gift an editor can bestow, confidence to go on writing. An agent was hardly necessary, but Doe Coover nevertheless offered her constant friendship, as well as some contract amendments.

My deepest debt, and the most difficult to acknowledge, is to my wife, Catherine Foote. I would like to avoid all the usual thanks that authors offer to their spouses: I share their embarrassment at recollecting how much writing a book demands from one's partner. So let me first thank Cathie as a colleague. The stories she has brought back from her own research on bereaved parents and her personal and clinical sensitivity to these stories have given me what sense I have of listening to the ill. And for all that the writing of this book has taken from her, both from our relationship and from her pursuit of her own work, I am at once sorry and grateful, that combination being the least of the oxymorons that hold together this fragile but encompassing marriage.

Finally, because my writing is always an attempt to leave behind traces of myself for my daughters, I thank them for being just who they are: Kate Libbey Frank and Stewart Hamilton-Frank.

One

When Bodies Need Voices

"The destination and map I had used to navigate before were no longer useful." These words were in a letter describing chronic fatigue syndrome. Judith Zaruches wrote of how, after an illness that is never really finished, she "needed . . . to think differently and construct new perceptions of my relationship to the world."[1]

Serious illness is a loss of the "destination and map" that had previously guided the ill person's life: ill people have to learn "to think differently." They learn by hearing themselves tell their stories, absorbing others' reactions, and experiencing their stories being shared. Judith's story not only stated her need for a new map and destination; her letter itself was an experimental performance of the different thinking she called for. Through the story she was telling me, her new map was already taking shape.

Even though we did not know each other, Judith needed to write to me—she had read my own story of cancer and seen a video tape of a lecture I gave—for me to witness her story and her personal change. As she told me her story, she discovered "new perceptions of [her] relationship to the world." That my response would only come later, in another letter, perhaps made it easier. Seeing herself write, like hearing herself speak, was the major threshold.

Judith's distinctiveness as a storyteller is her illness. Illness was not just the topic of her story; it was the condition of her telling that story. Her story was not just *about* illness. The story was told *through* a wounded body. The stories that ill people tell come out of their bodies. The body sets in motion the need for new stories when its disease disrupts the old stories. The body, whether still diseased or recovered, is simultaneously cause, topic, and instrument of whatever new stories are told.[2] These embodied stories have two sides, one personal and the other social.

The *personal* issue of telling stories about illness is to give voice to the body, so that the changed body can become once again familiar in these stories. But as the language of the story seeks to make the body familiar, the body eludes language. To paraphrase Martin Buber, the body "does not use speech, yet begets it."[3] The ill body is certainly not mute—it speaks eloquently in pains and symptoms—but it is inarticulate. We must speak for the body, and such speech is quickly frustrated: speech presents itself as being about the body rather than of it. The body is often alienated, literally "made strange," as it is told in stories that are instigated by a need to make it familiar.

The alternative to this frustration is to reduce the body to being the mere topic of the story and thus to deny the story's primary condition: the teller has or has had a disease. That the teller's diseased body shapes the illness story should be self-evident. Only a caricature Cartesianism would imagine a head, compartmentalized away from the disease, talking about the sick body beneath it. The head is tied to that body through pathways that science is only beginning to comprehend, but the general principle is clear: the mind does not rest above the body but is diffused throughout it.[4]

But actually hearing traces of the body in the story is not easy. Observing what stories say *about* the body is a familiar sort of listening; describing stories as told *through* the body requires another level of attention. This book attempts to evoke this other level of attention: How can we make sense of illness stories as being told *through* the diseased body?

The ill body's articulation in stories is a personal task, but the stories told by the ill are also *social*. The obvious social aspect of stories is that they are told *to* someone, whether that other person is immediately present or not. Even messages in a bottle imply a potential reader. The less evident social aspect of stories is that people do not make up their stories by themselves. The shape of the telling is molded by all the rhetorical expectations that the storyteller has been internalizing ever since he first heard some relative describe an illness, or she saw her first television commercial for a non-prescription remedy, or he was instructed to "tell the doctor what hurts" and had to figure out *what* counted as the story that the doctor wanted to hear. From their families and friends, from the popular culture that surrounds them, and from the stories of other ill people, storytellers have learned formal structures of narrative, conventional metaphors and imagery, and standards of what is and is not appropriate to tell. Whenever a new story is told, these rhetorical expectations are reinforced in some ways, changed in others, and passed on to affect others' stories.[5]

A first topic of this book is the *need* of ill people to tell their stories, in order to construct new maps and new perceptions of their relationships to the world. A second topic is the *embodiment* of these stories: how they are told not just about the body but through it. A third topic is the times that stories are told in: how the social context affects which stories get told and how they are told. The central issue of context is the distinction between illness as experienced in modern versus postmodern times.

POSTMODERN ILLNESS

The prefix "post" is not quite right; I do not propose any strict periodization of the modern and the postmodern. I do believe that over a period of time, perhaps the last twenty years, how people think about themselves and their worlds has changed enough to deserve a label, and the most accepted label—increasingly diffused in journalism and popular culture—is postmodernism.[6] Because of the number of intellectual agendae that employ some version of this label, I prefer "postmodern times." The times that contemporary illness stories are told in, which are also the times I am writing in, have changed fairly recently.

Albert Borgmann's title *Crossing the Postmodern Divide*[7] provides a particularly useful metaphor. Journeys cross divides. Once on the other side, the traveler remains the same person, carrying the same baggage. But on the other side of certain divides, the traveler senses a new identity; that same baggage now seems useful for new purposes. Fundamental assumptions that give life its particular meaning have changed. Postmodernity is such a crossing, occurring when the same ideas and actions are overlaid with different meanings. Sometimes these differences of having crossed the divide are clear, but more often they are subtle: things just feel different. Illness has come to feel different during the last twenty years, and today the sum of those differences can be labeled postmodernism. I make no attempt to define postmodernism; the utility of that term lies only in thick descriptions of the feel of the differences.

A useful, if simplified, evocation of the shift from the *premodern* experience of illness to modernity is provided by a North African woman quoted by Pierre Bourdieu in his anthropological research. That Bourdieu recorded this quotation from a living person is a reminder of the proximity and overlap of the premodern, modern, and postmodern. "In the old days," the woman said, "folk didn't know what illness was. They went to bed and they died. It's only nowadays that we've learned words like liver, lung, stomach, and I don't know what!"[8]

Of course premodern people had rich descriptors for disease and its remedies; ethnomedicine was and is highly specific. But I interpret the speaker's closing exclamation as indicating being overwhelmed: she literally doesn't know what. The specialized medical terms that the woman claims her people have only recently learned overwhelm her experience because they *come from elsewhere*. The shift to modernity crosses a divide into a medical culture that is foreign to this woman's experience of illness.

The *modern* experience of illness begins when popular experience is overtaken by technical expertise, including complex organizations of treatment. Folk no longer go to bed and die, cared for by family members and neighbors who have a talent for healing. Folk now go to paid professionals who reinterpret their pains as symptoms, using a specialized language that is unfamiliar and overwhelming. As patients, these folk accumulate entries on medical charts which in most instances they are neither able nor allowed to read; the chart becomes the official story of the illness. Other stories proliferate. Ill people tell family and friends versions of what the doctor said, and these others reply by telling experiences that seem to be similar: both experiences they have had themselves and ones heard from others. Illness becomes a *circulation of stories*, professional and lay, but not all stories are equal.

The story of illness that trumps all others in the modern period is the medical narrative. The story told by the physician becomes the one against which others are ultimately judged true or false, useful or not. I will discuss Talcott Parsons's theory of the "sick role" in later chapters.[9] What is relevant here is Parsons's observation, made about 1950, that a core social expectation of being sick is surrendering oneself to the care of a physician. I understand this obligation of seeking medical care as a *narrative surrender* and mark it as the central moment in modernist illness experience. The ill person not only agrees to follow physical regimens that are prescribed; she also agrees, tacitly but with no less implication, to tell her story in medical terms. "How are you?" now requires that personal feeling be contextualized within a secondhand medical report. The physician becomes the spokesperson for the disease, and the ill person's stories come to depend heavily on repetition of what the physician has said.

Times have come full circle from Bourdieu's North African informant when we read of a patient whose running joke with his surgeon involves reporting his symptoms in an overdone version of medical obscurity. For example, "If you will diligently investigate the pilar projections rising sparsely from the vertext of my cranial ossification, you will detect a macular callosity which may have malignant potential."[10] If modern medicine began when physicians asserted their authority as scientists by imposing specialized language on their patients' experiences, the postmodern divide is crossed when patients such as this one can mimic this language in a send-up of medicine that is shared with the physician. But lay familiarity with medical terms and techniques, even to the point of parody, is only one potential of the postmodern experience of illness.

The *postmodern* experience of illness begins when ill people recognize that more is involved in their experiences than the medical story can tell. The loss of a life's map and destination are not medical symptoms, at least until some psychiatric threshold is reached. The scope of modernist medicine—defined in practices ranging from medical school curricula to billing categories—does not include helping patients learn to think differently about their post-illness worlds and construct new relationships to those worlds. Yet people like Judith Zaruches express a self-conscious need to think differently.

Both the divide that was crossed from the premodern to the modern and that from modern to postmodern involve issues of voice. The woman reported by Bourdieu seems to perceive that medicine has taken away her voice: medicine assails her with words she does not want to know and leaves her not knowing what. But this woman does not perceive a need for what would now be called *her own voice,* a personal voice telling what illness has imposed on her and seeking to define for herself a new place in the world. What is distinct in postmodern times is people feeling a need for a voice they can recognize as their own.

This sense of need for a personal voice depends on the availability of the means—the rhetorical tools and cultural legitimacy—for expressing this voice. *Postmodern times are when the capacity for telling one's own story is reclaimed.* Modernist medicine hardly goes away: the postmodern claim to one's own voice is halting, self-doubting, and often inarticulate, but such claims have enough currency for illness to take on a different feel.

Voices tell stories. Stories are premodern; Bourdieu's informant suggests that the coming of modern medicine took away a capacity for experiencing illness in her folk's traditional stories. In the modern period the medical story has pride of place. Other stories become, as non-medical healers are called, "alternative," meaning secondary. The postmodern divide is crossed when people's own stories are no longer told as secondary but have their own primary importance.[11] Illness elicits more than fitting the body into traditional community expectations or surrendering the body to professional medicine, though both community traditions and professional medicine remain. Postmodern illness is an experience, a reflection on body, self, and the destination that life's map leads to.

The Remission Society

The possibility, even the necessity, of ill people telling their own stories has been set in place by the same modernist medicine that cannot contain these stories. At the end of the story that I wrote about my own experience of having cancer, I used the term "remission society" to describe all those people who, like me, were effectively well but could never be considered cured.[12] These people are all around, though often invisible. A man standing behind me in an airport security check announces that he has a pacemaker; suddenly his invisible "condition" becomes an issue. Once past the metal detector, his "remission" status disappears into the background.

Members of the remission society include those who have had almost any cancer, those living in cardiac recovery programs, diabetics, those whose allergies and environmental sensitivities require dietary and other self-monitoring, those with prostheses and mechanical body regulators, the chronically ill, the disabled, those "recovering" from abuses and addictions, and for all these people, the families that share the worries and daily triumph of staying well.

Cathy Pearse writes in middle-age about having a bleeding cerebral aneurysm—a stroke—when she was twenty.[13] During the operation, a cranial nerve was damaged. She still suffers from double vision, which she reports is "an ever present reminder" of her near-death experience. Her body is now beginning to feel the long-term effects of muscle asymmetry and favoring her "good side." But her illness history would be invisible to most people she meets, and she is long since considered "cured" by medicine. Cathy is a member of the remission society. Years after her hospitalization and treatment, she can still describe what happened in exquisite detail; she recalls the hurt caused by a nurse's casual comment as if it had been spoken yesterday. She refers to being a "recovered stroke patient" as one aspect of her "ethnicity," a word suggesting an irrevocable identity.

The physical existence of the remission society is modern: the technical achievements of modernist medicine make these lives possible. But people's self-consciousness of what it means to live in the wake of illness is postmodern. In modernist thought people are well *or* sick. Sickness and wellness shift definitively as to which is foreground and which is background at any given moment. In the remission society the foreground and background of sickness and health constantly shade into each other. Instead of a static picture on the page where light is separated from dark, the image is like a computer graphic where one shape is constantly in process of becoming the other.

Parsons's modernist "sick role" carries the expectation that ill people get well, cease to be patients, and return to their normal obligations. In the remission society people return, but obligations are never again what used to be normal. Susan Sontag's metaphor of illness as travel is more subtle than Parsons's sick role. We are each citizens of two kingdoms, Sontag writes, the kingdom of the well and that of the sick. "Although we all prefer to use only the good passport, sooner or later each of us is obliged, at least for a spell, to identify ourselves as citizens of that other place."[14] Sontag's notion of dual citizenship suggests a separation of these two kingdoms. The remission society is left to be either a demilitarized zone in between them, or else it is a secret society within the realm of the healthy.

To adapt Sontag's metaphor, members of the remission society do not use one passport *or* the other. Instead they are on permanent visa status, that visa requiring periodic renewal. The triumph of modernist medicine is to allow increasing numbers of people who would have been dead to enjoy this visa status, living in the world of the healthy even if always subject to expulsion. The problem for these people is that modernist medicine lacked a story appropriate to the experience it was setting in place. People like Judith Zaruches were left needing a new map for their lives.

The postmodernity of the remission society is more than a self-consciousness that has not been routinely available to the ill. Many members of the remission society feel a need to claim their visa status in an active voice. Those who work to express this voice are not only postmodern but, more specifically, *post-colonial* in their construction of self. Just as political and economic colonialism took over geographic areas, modernist medicine claimed the body of its patient as its territory, at least for the duration of the treatment. "When we're admitted to a hospital or even visiting a doctor," writes Dan Gottlieb, who as a quadriplegic has extensive experience with such visits, "the forms ask for 'Patient Name.' We stop being people and start being patients. . . . Our identity as people and the world we once knew both are relinquished; we become their patients and we live in their hospital."[15] Gottlieb's anger reflects a widespread resentment against medical colonization.

For those whose diseases are cured, more or less quickly and permanently, medical colonization is a temporary indignity. This colonization becomes an issue in the remission society when some level of treatment extends over the rest of a person's life, whether as periodic check-ups or as memories. The least form of treatment, periodic check-ups, are not "just" monitoring. "The fear comes and goes," writes Elizabeth Tyson, a breast cancer survivor, "but twice a year, at checkup time, it's ferocious."[16] For the person being checked, these check-ups represent the background of illness shading back into the foreground. Even for those whose visa is stamped expeditiously, the reality of lacking permanent citizenship is reaffirmed.

Colonization was central to the achievement of modernist medicine. Claudine Herzlich and Janine Pierret describe the "sick person" emerging as a recognizable social type in the early modern period, during the eighteenth century. The condition necessary for the emergence of this type was that "the diversity of suffering be reduced by a unifying general view, which is precisely that of clinical medicine."[17] This reducing of the particular to the general provided for scientific achievements, but the clinical reduction created a benevolent form of colonialism.

The ill person who plays out Parsons's sick role accepts having the particularity of his individual suffering reduced to medicine's general view. Modernity did not question this reduction because its benefits were immediate and its cost was not yet apparent. The colonization of experience was judged worth the cure, or the attempted cure. But illnesses have shifted from the acute to the chronic, and self-awareness has shifted. The post-colonial ill person, living with illness for the long term, wants her own suffering recognized in its individual particularity; "reclaiming" is the relevant postmodern phrase.

In postmodern times more and more people, with varying degrees of articulation and action, express suspicion of medicine's reduction of their suffering to its general unifying view. Members of the remission society, who know medicine from the inside out, question their place in medical narratives. What they question can be clarified by drawing an analogy to people who were politically colonized. Gayatri Chakravorty Spivak speaks of colonized people's efforts "to see how the master texts need us in [their] construction . . . without acknowledging that need."[18] What do the master texts of medicine need but not acknowledge?

I met a man who had a cancer of the mouth that required extensive reconstructive surgery to his jaw and face. His treatment had been sufficiently extraordinary for his surgeon to have published a medical journal article about it, complete with pictures showing the stages of the reconstructive process.

When he told me about the article and offered to show it to me, I imagined the article might actually be about *him:* his suffering throughout this mutilating, if life-saving, ordeal. As I looked at the article I realized his name was not mentioned. Probably the surgeon and the journal would have considered it unethical to name him, even though pictures of the man were shown. Thus in "his" article he was systematically ignored as anyone—actually anything—other than a body. But for medical purposes it was not his article at all; it was his surgeon's article. This is exactly the colonization that Spivak speaks of: the master text of the medical journal article needs the suffering person, but the individuality of that suffering cannot be acknowledged.

Most ill people remain willing to continue to play the medical "patient" game by modernist rules without question, and almost all do so when required. But post-colonial members of the remission society are demanding, in various and often frustrated ways, that medicine recognize its need for them. Refusing to be reduced to "clinical material" in the construction of the medical text, they are claiming voices.

Because illness, following medicine, is effectively privatized, this demand for voice rarely achieves a collective force. Feminist health activists are a major exception. Susan Bell writes about the attempts by members of the Cambridge Women's Community Health Center (WCHC) to change the role played by women who were recruited by Harvard Medical School to serve as paid "pelvic models" for medical students to learn to perform gynecological examinations.[19] Bell tells of the women's escalating demands to participate in a full teaching role rather than serve as inert bodies to be taught upon. Women negotiated for their own class time with medical students, they sought to demonstrate how women could perform their own gynecological examinations using a mirror, and they injected political issues into the medical curriculum.

The medical school finally rejected WCHC demands that teaching be limited to women (since the experience of being examined should be, in principle, reciprocal), that non-student hospital personnel and other consumers be included in the teaching sessions, and that more political discussion contextualize the medical teaching. The specifics of the WCHC demands are less important than their basic post-colonial stance: women wanted to have their necessity acknowledged in the construction of medical knowledge and practice. They claimed an active voice in that knowledge and practice.[20]

Post-colonialism in its most generalized form is the demand to speak rather than being spoken for and to represent oneself rather than being represented or, in the worst cases, rather than being effaced entirely. But in postmodern times pressures on clinical practice, including the cost of physicians' time and ever greater use of technologies, mean less time for patients to speak.[21] People then speak elsewhere. The post-colonial impulse is acted out less in the clinic than in stories that members of the remission society tell each other about their illnesses.[22]

The post-colonial stance of these stories resides not in the content of what they say about medicine. Rather the new feel of these stories begins in how often medicine and physicians do *not* enter the stories. Postmodern illness stories are told so that people can place themselves outside the "unifying general view." For people to move their stories outside the professional purview involves a profound assumption of personal responsibility. In Parsons's sick role the ill person as patient was responsible only for getting well; in the remission society, the post-colonial ill person takes responsibility for what illness means in his life.

POSTMODERN RESPONSIBILITY

Anthony Giddens describes the contemporary self "as a reflexive project, for which the individual is responsible."[23] The notion of the self as a reflexive project echoes Socrates' advocacy of the examined life, but Socrates was speaking to an elite, and how far he advocated *changing* one's life as a result of self-examination is debatable. The modernist responsibility that Giddens refers to has its epigram in the famous line of the poet Rilke, "You must change your life."[24] Modernity is premised on people's capacity to change their lives; philosophical self-examination becomes a practical challenge. Giddens's "reflexive project" describes people taking up Rilke's challenge.

In postmodern times the reflexive project of self can yield two different sorts of identities, contrasted by Zygmunt Bauman to suggest developments that are either more or less responsible. The line of self-development that I understand as less responsible gives rise to what Bauman calls "'momentary' identities, identities 'for today', until-further-notice identities."[25] Such a self is primarily responsible to itself; its responsibilities are limited to the sphere of its own perceived self-interest. This sphere may include others, but these others are included "until further notice."

The alternative form of postmodern self—though it is hardly unique to postmodern times—is described in Bauman's summary of the moral philosophy of Emmanuel Levinas: "I being *for* the Other, I bearing *responsibility* for the Other."[26] Since defining the self in terms of responsibility for the other is the core ethical impulse in most religions, the parable of the Good Samaritan being one of the most succinct examples, what news is there in Bauman's and Levinas's revival of this idea? One response is that so long as practice continues to fall short of the ideal, the ideal must be reaffirmed in the idiom of each age.

A stronger response is that Levinas means something different from how the Samaritan ideal is conventionally interpreted. Living *for* the other is not, as Levinas describes it, an act of exemplary goodness. Persons live *for* others because their own lives as humans require living that way. The self is understood as coming to be human in relation to others, and the self can only continue to be human by living *for* the Other. Bauman concludes his book with a discussion of the ethics of dying for another person; the self that is willing to sacrifice itself for another could not be further removed from the "until-further-notice" sense of responsibility.

For present purposes, however—and I return to Levinas in chapter 9—the importance of Bauman and Levinas is that in secular modernist culture the ideal of living *for* the other has been sufficiently lost that redefining it does constitute news. Bauman demonstrates how the sense of responsibility for the specific other person—as opposed to collective others—was a casualty of modernity. An understanding of why modern medicine has limited the concept of responsibility as it has, and of how sociology has justified this limitation, can be derived from his work.

Parsons's sick role articulated the modernist requirement that ill persons delegate responsibility for their health to physicians; illness responsibility is reduced to patient compliance. Physicians as described in Parsons's sociology are in turn responsible more to professional codes than to individual patients. According to modernist universalism, the greatest responsibility to *all* patients is achieved when the professional places adherence to the profession before the particular demands of any individual patient.

Such professionalism—paradigmatic of modernity—is responsible less to individual people than to truth, understood on several levels: the factual truth of medical science, the beneficent truth of institutional management in the hospital, and ultimately the political truth of administering people's welfare, which Michel Foucault calls biopolitics.[27] Modernity accepted these truths, and this acceptance required the patient's narrative surrender to medicine.

These modernist truths remain the basis of professional practice even on this side of the postmodern divide, and popular demand for that practice increases. The prospect of economic necessity requiring explicit rationing of health care provokes fear in many people. The ambivalence on this side of the divide is that, simultaneous with increased demand, confidence in the possibility of truth delivering on its promises has faded. The same people who one moment are fearful that their health care will be rationed may, in the next moment, attend a pro-choice meeting on euthanasia and speak of their fear of "dying on a machine." People still need their specific professionals, but professions as a group are regarded with increasing cynicism. Strains in lay/professional relations reflect not only conflicts of expectations between these groups, but conflicts within each group's expectations as well.[28]

Ill people still surrender their bodies to medicine, but increasingly they try to hold onto their own stories. Refusing narrative surrender becomes one specific activity of reflexive monitoring, and thus an exercise of responsibility.

The status of personal responsibility is a central moral issue for postmodernity. Bauman's description of the momentary identity that holds itself to no particular standard expresses the cynical response to the demise of truth. An alternative was expressed at the beginning of the century by William James, whose prescient modernism may already have crossed the postmodern divide. One of James's letters is the finest epigram I have found to the particular assumption of responsibility that is equally a potential of postmodern times:

I am convinced that the desire to formulate truths is a
virulent disease. It has contracted an alliance lately in
me with a feverish personal ambition, which I never
had before, and which I recognize as an unholy thing
in such a connection. I actually dread to die until I
have settled the Universe's hash in one more
book. . . ! Childish idiot—as if formulas about the
Universe could ruffle its majesty and as if the
commonsense world and its duties were not eternally
the really real.[29]

Like a good postmodernist, James rejects truth, but he does
so on moral grounds that other aspects of postmodernity often
negate.

James is concerned about his own corruption by the "unholy" alliance of truth and personal ambition. His rejection of
the attempt to state universal truth—the stuff that could settle
the Universe's hash—seems a necessary prerequisite to an enhanced sense of responsibility. In place of universal truth James
affirms the "really real" of "the commonsense world and its duties." I read that last word, *duties*, as the strongest in his confes-
sion.

Ill people's storytelling is informed by a sense of responsibility to the commonsense world and represents one way of
living *for* the other. People tell stories not just to work out
their own changing identities, but also to guide others who
will follow them. They seek not to provide a map that can
guide others—each must create his own—but rather to witness the experience of reconstructing one's own map. Witnessing is one duty to the commonsensical and to others.

The idea of telling one's story as a responsibility to the commonsense world reflects what I understand as the core morality of the postmodern. Storytelling is *for* an other just as much
as it is for oneself. In the reciprocity that is storytelling, the

so: guide (more than witness)

testimoned

teller offers herself as guide to the other's self-formation. The other's receipt of that guidance not only recognizes but *values* the teller. The moral genius of storytelling is that each, teller and listener, enters the space of the story *for* the other. Telling stories in postmodern times, and perhaps in all times, attempts to change one's own life by affecting the lives of others. Thus all stories have an element of *testimony,* and the particular testimony of illness stories will be developed in later chapters.

✿ ✿ ✿

Telling stories of illness is the attempt, instigated by the body's disease, to give a voice to an experience that medicine cannot describe. This voice is embodied in a specific person, but it is equally social, taking its speech from the postmodern times we live in. The voice of the ill person is made possible by modernist medicine, but it cannot be contained within modernist assumptions, particularly those about medical professional dominance and the narrative surrender this dominance requires. A divide has been crossed into new territory, the postmodern, and we know this crossing by the new voices that are heard.

As a post-colonial voice, the storyteller seeks to reclaim her own experience of suffering. As she seeks to turn that suffering into testimony, the storyteller engages in moral action. The themes of body, voice, and illness culminate in the ethics made uniquely possible in postmodern times. Postmodernity is not often described in ethical terms, and when it is, the assessment is usually that "postmodern ethics" is an oxymoron.

In a chapter entitled "The Post-Modern Void," Alan Wolfe summarizes the intellectual trends of postmodernity as indicating that "nothing is eternal, all value is relative, meaning is self-referential, and the sacred is little more than an ideological construct imposed by those who hold power over those who lack it."[30] Wolfe certainly assesses one aspect of postmodernity correctly. But in postmodern times, to seek the eternal, the valued, and the sacred in intellectual trends is to look in the wrong place.

Postmodernity has its distinctive ethics, but these must be sought in the everyday personal struggles of people like Judith Zaruches, Cathy Pearse, and Dan Gottlieb, who are trying to make moral sense of their own suffering and who are witnesses to sufferings that go beyond their own. William James's direction to attend to the commonsense world and its duties still informs the task of the intellectual in postmodern times. The circle of witnesses includes not just ill persons and those who care for them, but the intellectuals who observe these people and their struggles. In these observations, postmodern intellectuals can affirm what is eternal, valuable, meaningful, and sacred.

Wolfe's observation of "the post-modern void" is a welcome reminder of the risk of our times. Just as James felt personally at risk from his "feverish personal ambition," the postmodern intellectual is at risk. James feared his ambition to settle "the Universe's hash." To settle the Universe's hash is to place oneself outside the vulnerability and contingency that being in the Universe involves. The intellectual infected with such an ambition ceases to think of himself as a body, thus disclaiming the vulnerability that bodies share. Ceasing to think of oneself as a body severs a connection that is fundamental to thinking of oneself as a person who exists *for* other people. Social science—or any academic and professional discipline that observes and attends the ill—must accept responsibility for its observations as acts of witness that commit the scientist as a person.[31]

The premise of this book is that responsibility begins and ends with the body. Both observation and witness begin with a body, and both commit that body. I concluded an earlier review article by calling for an ethics of the body.[32] Such a project is too large for one lifetime, much less one book. No one can settle the body's hash, but I hope the present book begins to make good on that call. Postmodern times are a void only if people cease to fill those times with meaning.

ABOUT THIS BOOK

A constant theme of social theory is contingency, interpreted as the problem of how stable a course of action can be when this action depends on, but cannot control, some other action. I have made the body's contingency—how much any of us can depend on our bodies—a major theme below. So perhaps it is fitting that the materials forming the basis of this book were collected through contingent circumstances.

I began academic life as a medical sociologist and then gave it up because I had trouble gaining access to what interested me most, the direct experiences of ill persons. After a decade of pursuing other topics, I returned—or *was* returned—to illness experience. In 1985 I suffered a heart attack (ventricular tachycardia) as a result of a viral infection. It was a highly contingent heart attack, I was told, dependent on a virus that might have acted otherwise. Just over a year later I was feeling fully recovered when I began to notice the symptoms that eventually proved to be testicular cancer (a seminoma tumor). A year after I had ended treatment myself, my mother-in-law, Laura Foote, came out of cancer remission for the last time.

In 1989 I wrote about these events in what might be called an analytic memoir, *At the Will of the Body: Reflections on Illness*, published in 1991. Since 1992 that book has been the basis of continuing personal encounters, letters, phone calls, conferences, and lectures that have kept me in contact with individual ill persons and support groups, as well as nursing, chaplain, administrative, and medical groups.

I have tried to tell medical residents what it is like to be seriously ill, my talks usually taking place during the lunch break while they gulp down the pizza, soda, and cookies provided by

social rhetoric of illness

drug companies expressing their usual commitment to health. I have listened to what medical students hope to become as physicians and to what they fear may happen to them in practice. In other hospitals, in what seems like another world, I have listened as a support group of parents began their meeting by each saying the name of their child who had died and adding, if emotion allowed further speech, what the cause of death had been. When I was introduced as the evening's speaker, I wondered what I could possibly tell them about suffering. These personal experiences frame this book.

My direct experiences in the world of illness are complemented by reading many published and unpublished illness stories.[33] The published works are particularly important to this book because, being published, they are easily quoted: readers can reread the stories for themselves. Published stories also have a particular influence: they affect how others tell their stories, creating the social rhetoric of illness. But published materials have their problems. There can be no pretense of a "sample" of this writing, both because there is so much written and because illness figures variously in many different memoirs. What counts as an illness story is by no means clear.[34]

A more substantive problem is the appropriate suspicion about how any published account may have been shaped by editorial forces that the author might have wanted to resist.[35] I know this shaping occurs; I know that even when I have talked to a book's editors I can never be sure how any particular account was shaped; yet I continue to believe that published stories are "true." The truth of experience is malleable.

My own experience of publishing my story can serve to illustrate the complex interactions of storytelling and experience. By the time *At the Will of the Body* was ready for publication, I wondered if I had compromised too much and if the story was still "mine." I had written every word, but as editorial advice accumulated, I was less than confident whose voice was being written. Now I can hardly remember what those compromises were: either the book has become my experience, or my experience always was the book. Thus I return to my claim that even edited stories remain true. The truth of stories is not only what *was* experienced, but equally what *becomes* experience in the telling and its reception.

The stories we tell about our lives are not necessarily those lives as they were lived, but these stories become our experience of those lives. A published narrative of an illness is not the illness itself, but it can become the experience of the illness. The social scientific notion of reliability—getting the same answer to the same question at different times—does not fit here. Life moves on, stories change with that movement, and experience changes. Stories are true to the flux of experience, and the story affects the direction of that flux.

If calling stories true requires some category of stories called false, I confess to being unsure what a "false" personal account would be. I have read personal accounts I considered evasive, but that evasion *was* their truth. The more reconstructed the story, the more powerful the truth of the *desire* for what is being told, as the corrected version of what was lived. Hearing the desire in the story takes me back to the need for a different level of attention to stories.

A final influence on this book is that as I write I am in the middle of my three-year term as editor of the "Case Stories" series in the professional journal *Second Opinion: Health, Faith, Ethics.*[36] My commitment in the series is to publish first-person accounts of illness experience. Each "story" has two commentators who ostensibly write in a "professional" voice, but like many distinctions in postmodern times, the first and third-person voices seem hard to separate. Faced with first-person stories, the commentators tell their own stories. At issue in the commentaries, as throughout this book, is the question of what can be said about a story of primary witness, and to what extent the story has to be left to speak for itself.

My most provocative, and often troubling, editorial task has been requesting revisions to people's stories. I recognize that in asking authors to revise their stories, I may be asking them to revise their experiences. Recently an author, Richard Morgan, was asked by one of the journal's manuscript reviewers to provide more medical detail in his story. In response, he subpoenaed and read his medical chart. He told me he then understood, for the first time, what had happened to him during his surgery and hospitalization. Perhaps he did; or perhaps he now has a new story, no more or less true to his experience than his old one, but partially instigated by the editorial machinery. My own experience of reading stories at all stages of editorial review has formed the ideas in this book, not least by affecting how I read published accounts that I have not had an editorial hand in.

My objective with these eclectic materials—stories heard in person, read in print, and watched being shaped for publication—is to develop a practice for doing what I heard an anthropologist recommend while attempting to explain a native oral tradition to a white audience: "You have to learn to think *with* stories."[37] Not think about stories, which would be the usual phrase, but think with them. To think about a story is to reduce it to content and then analyze that content. Thinking with stories takes the story as already complete; there is no going beyond it. To think with a story is to experience it affecting one's own life and to find in that effect a certain truth of one's life. Thus in this book people's illness stories are not "data" to support various propositions that I advance. Instead, the stories are the materials that I use to model theorizing— and living—with stories.

My project in clinical ethics is to move ethicists and practitioners in the direction of thinking *with* stories: to help professionals to recognize ill persons' stories and all they represent. The complementary project in social science might be called a sociology of witness. I seek to situate both clinical ethics and social science within a more general ethics of the body. Such an ethics develops terms of responsibility to the stories told *through* suffering bodies. Being responsible to these stories, thinking with them, depends on telling certain stories over and over, hearing different nuances of potential meaning as the story is told in different circumstances and at different ages of our lives. Thus in this book I return to comparatively few illness stories.

Thinking with stories is not nostalgia for a premodern oral culture. On our present side of the postmodern divide any thinking with stories carries the baggage of modernity. Thus I retell stories and then, like a good modernist, place them into analytical frameworks. My defense for this procedure is that in times when we have lost the premodern feel for stories, heuristic frameworks can help to hear them. Frameworks can disentangle types of narratives; they can help in recognizing what basic life concerns are being addressed and how the story proclaims a certain relation of the body to the world. The frameworks are not the truth of the stories, which is how modernism often presented its typologies. The frameworks I present are only a means of heightening attention to stories that are their own truth.

Thinking with stories ultimately requires a highly personal sedimentation of experience: living with the stories and having them shape perceptions of various experiences over time. I began reading other people's illness stories just after I was ill myself, and the stories in which I most often anchor my thoughts remain those I read first, just because I have lived with them the longest and had them recur to me in the most varied situations. Some more recent stories may be "better" to make certain points, but stories take time to become mine. My ambition for this book is to facilitate each reader's own sedimentation, but that process can only occur in each reader's own experience, and experience takes time to sediment.

After having cancer I attempted to read some of the professional literature describing the experience I had gone through. I found the language too distant from the immediacy of embodied suffering that I had recently experienced. In Spivak's terms, the professional text needed my body, but it could not acknowledge that need.[38] Now I sense this book about others' stories becoming too analytical, too distant from embodied experience, too modernist in its rationalization of experience. But following James, I seek not to settle the hash of even that small corner of the universe called human illness in late twentieth century North America. Rather I want only to affirm the commonsense world and its duties.

One of our most difficult duties as human beings is to listen to the voices of those who suffer. The voices of the ill are easy to ignore, because these voices are often faltering in tone and mixed in message, particularly in their spoken form before some editor has rendered them fit for reading by the healthy. These voices bespeak conditions of embodiment that most of us would rather forget our own vulnerability to. Listening is hard, but it is also a fundamental moral act; to realize the best potential in postmodern times requires an ethics of listening. I hope to show that in listening for the other, we listen for ourselves. The moment of witness in the story crystallizes a mutuality of need, when each is *for* the other.

Two

The Body's Problems with Illness

The body is not mute, but it is inarticulate; it does not use speech, yet begets it. The speech that the body begets includes illness stories; the problem of hearing these stories is to hear the body speaking in them. People telling illness stories do not simply describe their sick bodies; their bodies give their stories their particular shape and direction. People certainly talk about their bodies in illness stories; what is harder to hear in the story is the body creating the person.

Hearing the body in the speech it begets is never an easy task. Although the body has been a frequent topic of social science in recent years, no satisfactory solution has been found to avoid reducing the body to a thing that is described. Arthur and Joan Kleinman critique social science's limited concern "with *what* the body's cultural form means and *why* its representation differs in different epochs and among different people." The body becomes an object existing in different cultures, another cultural artifact to be described. Such writing ignores the complex mutual relation between the body and culture, what the Kleinmans call infolding and outfolding.

Referring to their own field, the Kleinmans write what should become a maxim for any students of the body: "A medical anthropology unable or unwilling to examine how culture infolds into the body (and, reciprocally, how bodily processes outfold into social space) is not very likely to get far in conceptualization and empirical study of the sociopolitical roots of illness or the cultural sources of healing."[1]

The Kleinmans' solution to this problem is to invoke the language of medical symptoms. Their empirical analysis of contemporary China uses symptoms to read how bodies have recorded the effects of a half century of trauma, from the revolutions preceding World War II through Tiananmen Square. They write: "Symptoms of social suffering, and the transformations they undergo, *are* the cultural forms of lived experience. They are lived memories. [Symptoms] bridge social institutions and the body-self" (716). Bodily symptoms are the infolding of cultural traumas into the body. As these bodies continue to live and to create history, these symptoms outfold into the social space of that history. The Kleinmans provide one of the most sophisticated analyses of the interweaving of bodies, cultures, and lives, and the limitations of their efforts to hear the body speaking reveal the dilemma that every such attempt, including my own, must struggle with.

In order to hear bodies speak, the Kleinmans have to express bodies in a language of symptoms. As descriptors of the body, the language of symptoms is not transparent; as suggested in chapter 1, it imposes its own "general unifying view" on bodies. But this language is as good as any other: the speech that the body begets *always* imposes itself upon the body. The issue then becomes what language I will now impose on ill bodies, in order to show "how bodily processes outfold" through their stories, as well as how, in these stories, "culture infolds into the body."

I begin with some basic questions about how to act as the embodied being that the Kleinmans call a "body-self." During illness, people who have always *been* bodies have distinctive problems *continuing* to be bodies, particularly continuing to be the same sorts of bodies they have been. The body's problems during illness are not new; being a body always involves certain problems. Illness requires new and more self-conscious solutions to these general problems. In earlier writing I have proposed four general problems of embodiment: control, body-relatedness, other-relatedness, and desire.[2] These problems, developed in detail in the rest of this chapter, are *general* body problems. One way or another, everyone has been resolving—if never finally "solving"—these problems throughout her life.

Each body problem is a problem of *action:* to act, a body-self must achieve some working resolution to each problem. The ways that a body-self responds to each problem are presented as a continuum or range of possible responses; thus four problems yield four continua. I emphasize that each range of possible actions, while it looks on paper like a dichotomy, is in reality a continuum of responses.

Within the matrix of these four continua, I generate four ideal typical bodies: the disciplined body, the mirroring body, the dominating body, and the communicative body. Each of these types is described in the sections that follow. The language I will use to talk about bodies thus consists of these four problems of action, the four continua of responses to these problems, and the four ideal typical bodies.

This language is an imposition on bodies; real people are not ideal types. Ideal types are puppets: theoretical constructions designed to describe some empirical *tendency.*[3] Actual body-selves represent distinctive mixtures of ideal types. If in later chapters the four ideal types of bodies prove inadequate to what is "really real" in the stories, this inadequacy is not a problem; the theory is doing what it is supposed to do. As James understood, the "really real" does not exist in order to be theorized. But theory is still useful in approaching the bewildering particularity of that really real. Ideal types provide a reflexive medium, a language, for talking about what is particular in real bodies.

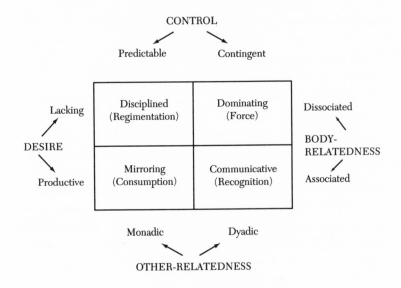

BODY PROBLEMS

The Problem of Control

Everyone must ask in any situation, Can I reliably predict how my body will function; can I *control* its functioning?

People define themselves in terms of their body's varying capacity for control. So long as these capacities are predictable, control as an action problem does not require self-conscious monitoring. But disease itself is a loss of predictability, and it causes further losses: incontinence, shortness of breath or memory, tremors and seizures, and all the other "failures" of the sick body. Some ill people adapt to these contingencies easily; others experience a crisis of control. Illness is about learning to live with lost control.

The question of control suggests that the body is lived along a continuum from the *predictability* that may reach its highest expression in ballet and gymnastics to *contingency* at the other end. Contingency is the body's condition of being subject to forces that cannot be controlled. The infantile body is contingent: burping, spitting, and defecating according to its own internal needs and rhythms. Society expects nothing more, and infants are afforded some period to acquire control. When adult bodies lose control, they are expected to attempt to regain it if possible, and if not then at least to conceal the loss as effectively as possible.

A man described to me the social problems he experienced when he lost bladder control following surgery for prostate cancer. He was expected to conceal the contingency of his bladder; stains and smells are stigmatizing. But he also found that sales people in home-care stores were unwilling to discuss incontinence products with him, in part, it seemed to him, because he was male (incontinence is, demographically, more a female problem) and perhaps also because he was younger than social stereotypes of incontinence allowed.

Erving Goffman's classic work on stigma shows that society demands a considerable level of body control from its members; loss of this control is stigmatizing, and special work is required to manage the lack of control.[4] Stigma, Goffman points out, is embarrassing, not just for the stigmatized person but for those who are confronted with the stigma and have to react to it. Thus the work of the stigmatized person is not only to avoid embarrassing himself by being out of control in situations where control is expected. The person must also avoid embarrassing others, who should be protected from the specter of lost body control.

Stigma imposed on the ill represents social ambivalence over what kind of contingency illness is. Parsons's sick-role theory states the dominant medical ideology that persons are not responsible for being ill, but Goffman shows that they are responsible for how they present themselves and manifest the signs of their illness. While society remains ambivalent, a post-colonial affirmation of stigma has emerged. Members of Alcoholics Anonymous become less anonymous when they display bumper stickers of AA slogans. Published illness stories that reveal a variety of bodily stigmas are another affirmation of being a stigmatized body-self.[5]

Goffman defined *passing* as keeping from public view a "spoiled identity" that was otherwise invisible. When I wear the lapel pin of my own cancer support group I am doing a kind of reverse passing, proclaiming my identity to be spoiled even though I could easily pass. This behavior would fit the generic type "coming out," which is distinctively postmodern. But the membership pin or bumper sticker also proclaims a person who is "doing something" about a contingency that is thus defined as not entirely contingent. This "doing something" about contingency is meta-control. Turning illness into story is a kind of meta-control, although meta-control is only one reason for storytelling.

A body's place on the continuum of control depends not only on the physiological possibility of predictability or contingency, but also on how the person chooses to interpret this physiology. The flesh cannot be denied, but bodies are more than mere corporeality. As body-selves, people interpret their bodies and make choices: the person can either seek perfected levels of predictability, at whatever cost, or can accept varying degrees of contingency. Most people do both, and strategies vary as to what is sought to be controlled, where, and how.

How any individual responds to lost predictability is woven into the dense fabric of how the other action problems of the body are managed, since the same illness provokes crises in these other dimensions as well.

Body-Relatedness[6]

Is my body the flesh that "I," the cognitive, ethereal I, only happen to inhabit, or is whatever "I" am only to be found as my body? Do I *have* a body, or *am* I a body?[7]

A friend of mine had an inflammation of lymph nodes under his arms. Physicians did not find any disease (and the years proved them correct), but they advised him to check the swelling daily for any change, tenderness, or other symptom. He told me what he disliked was "having to be embodied," which I understood to mean having to attend to his body on a daily and intimate basis, taking this body seriously as having implications for who he was. He preferred, apparently, to get his body dressed as soon as possible and then regard "it" as disappeared within his clothes. He didn't like to eat, and liquids were consumed for the pleasure of that consumption, not in recognition of the body's needs. He represents the *dissociated* end of the continuum.

I myself tend toward the opposite end, choosing to live in a body that I am compulsively *associated* with. I believe I am what I eat. I do *tai chi* exercises in order to become more aware of my body's balance and tensions. I once saw enlargements of a slide of my recently drawn blood. I think about that blood: the red cells sometimes bonding together, the white cells eating bacteria, and even the odd cancer cells, whose presence is perfectly normal. I know who I am as much in that blood as in this writing or any other activity.

But bodies are not simply associated with or dissociated from. Here as elsewhere, the continuum is not really linear; in this case the quality of association changes.

Zygmunt Bauman points out a paradox of body association: the body, at least in the end that will come to us all, is the enemy of survival.[8] As long as the body is healthy and mortality is beyond the horizon of consciousness, associating the self with the body comes easily. The recognition of mortality complicates this association. Legend has it that Gautama who later became the Buddha left his palace and became an ascetic after seeing bodies that exemplified suffering, decay, and death. Until then he had been sheltered from such sights, and his association with his body was based on the illusion that bodies brought only gratification. When he learned what troubles the body is prone to, he dissociated himself from his body through asceticism.

The Buddha's later enlightenment included his renunciation of asceticism and ability to move back into his body. By then the quality of association changed for him. His body association was no longer either tacit or hedonistic but became a moral choice to accept his lot as a body prone to suffering. Some body association is simply naïve to suffering; another level of association accepts its mortality. In the really real, the continuum of body-relatedness is not linear but spirals.

Modernist medicine does much to discourage body association. Robert Zussman in his study of intensive care units quotes one physician: "I think you don't have to look at a patient here, basically. You don't have to examine a patient. . . . The numbers, I feel, they are more reliable."[9] Such physicians then teach their patients that with respect to how they feel, the numbers, or diagnostic images, or cardiac tracings, are more reliable. Most of us, sooner or later, go to the doctor to find out how we feel, our distrust of subjective feelings being a form of dissociation.

Many healers outside of orthodox medicine, whom I will call "alternatives" for convenience, practice teaching the patient refined sensitivity to how he feels, and teaching him to trust that feeling. The shift to alternative healing—survey data suggest that more visits are made to alternative practitioners than to orthodox physicians—is another indicator of crossing a postmodern divide. Again, the same baggage is brought over the divide: most people who visit alternative healers continue to see medical physicians.[10] But for people who are seeing an alternative healer, what it feels like to see the orthodox medical practitioners changes.

Other-Relatedness

What is my relationship, as a body, to other persons who are also bodies? How does our shared corporeality affect who we are, not only to each other, but more specifically *for* each other? Other-relatedness as an action problem is concerned with how the shared condition of being bodies becomes a basis of empathic relations among living beings. Albert Schweitzer expressed this concern in his phrase, the "brotherhood of those who bear the mark of pain."

In 1921, following both his first medical missionary expedition to Africa and a period of severe illness resulting from his internment as an enemy alien during World War I, Schweitzer wrote what became one of his most famous passages:

> Whoever among us has learned through personal
> experience what pain and anxiety really are must help
> to ensure that those out there who are in physical
> need obtain the same help that once came to him.
> He no longer belongs to himself alone; he has
> become the brother of all who suffer. It is this
> "brotherhood of those who bear the mark of pain"
> that demands humane medical services. . . . [11]

My term for the body's sense of this "brotherhood" is the *dyadic* body. Schweitzer's contemporary, Martin Buber, wrote of perceiving a tree that "it is bodied over against me and has to do with me, as I with it."[12] The dyadic relation is the recognition that even though the other is a body outside of mine, "over against me," this other *has to do with me, as I with it.*

Illness presents a particular opening to becoming a dyadic body, because the ill person is immersed in a suffering that is both wholly individual—my pain is mine alone—but also shared: the ill person sees others around her, before and after her, who have gone through this same illness and suffered their own wholly particular pains. She sees others who are pained by her pain. Storytelling is one medium through which the dyadic body both offers its own pain and receives the reassurance that others recognize what afflicts it. Thus storytelling is a privileged medium of the dyadic body.

At the opposite end of the other-relatedness continuum is the *monadic* body, understanding itself as existentially separate and alone. A 1991 film, *The Doctor*, shows William Hurt as a surgeon who has just been told he has cancer. His wife receives the news with a "we" statement about their ability as a couple to cope with whatever comes. He corrects her, saying that *he* alone has cancer. Many, like this character, choose the monadic body when faced with illness. That the character is a surgeon is an interesting comment on cultural perceptions of where medicine places bodies on the continuum from monadic to dyadic.

Medicine encourages monadic bodies in many ways. Hospitals treat patients in close enough proximity to each other to obviate any meaningful privacy, but at just enough distance to eliminate any meaningful contact. Some friendships are formed in waiting rooms and between roommates, but in my observations of cancer centers, most contact among patients is minimal and transitory. Patients relate individually to medical staff, not collectively among themselves, and this pattern of relating seems to result from how medical spaces are designed and how movement within them is orchestrated. Modernist administrative systems not only prefer the monadic body, but the disease model that grounds medical practice has little ability to admit any other concept of the body.[13]

The monadic body of medicine articulates well with modernist society's emphasis on individual achievement in education or in the marketplace. The dyadic body thus represents an ethical *choice* to place oneself in a different relationship to others. This choice is to be a body *for* other bodies.[14] Living for others means placing one's self and body within the "community of pain," to render Schweitzer's phrase contemporary.

Thus my continua are not only not linear, as the shifting nature of body association demonstrates; they are also ideal types of ethical *choices*. The choice to live as a dyadic body points toward an ethics of the body. Dyadic bodies exist *for* each other: they exist for the task of discovering what it means to live for other bodies. The dyadic body is a lived reality, not simply a conceptual ethical ideal. Schweitzer writes as one who dedicated his life, and body, to actualizing the ideal of the community of pain. But acting for the other cannot proceed apart from contemplative reflection on this action: Schweitzer took considerable time away from his medical work to continue to write.

Desire

What do I *want*, and how is this desire expressed *for* my body, *with* my body, and *through* my body?

My usage of desire has its conceptual roots in the psychoanalytic theory of Jacques Lacan.[15] Lacan places desire in a triad with need and demand. The need is fully corporeal and can be satisfied at that level. The baby needs milk or a dry diaper. The expression of the need is the demand, but the demand differs from the need itself: the baby's cry is not the same as its hunger or wetness. The demand's difference from the need enlarges the context: the demand asks for more than the need it seeks to express.

Desire is this quality of *more*. When the child asks for one more of whatever at bedtime—one more story, one more drink, one more hug—that displacement of each "more" by another expresses the desire in the demand. The parents' frustration is that when they fulfill the demand, the child remains unhappy. Desire, Lacan teaches, cannot be filled: there is always more.

I read expressions of this desire constantly in people's stories. Dan Wakefield, in his widely read spiritual autobiography, expresses Lacanian desire when he writes, "I wanted—needed, it felt like—*more.*"[16] Robert Coles reports a student's story about her mother's compulsive shopping; the terms are explicitly Lacanian: "Need was beside the point; she had everything. Desire was the point—to think of something she wanted. . . ."[17] Desire has to express itself as the demand for some object, but the object is not what is desired, any more than the child at bedtime desires what he demands. The point of desire is that the displacements never end: there is no final demand; desire is always wanting more.

Yet some bodies, particularly ill bodies, do cease desiring. The body's problem of desire generates a continuum between bodies that have come to *lack* desire and those that remain *productive* of desire. Illness often precipitates a condition of lacking desire. Stewart Alsop, dying of leukemia, writes of his approaching birthday that perhaps being sixty "is a good time to bow out."[18] This statement will receive full interpretation in a later chapter; I quote it here for its commonsense quality of resignation: desire is lacking.

Malcolm Diamond, writing about his reaction to the diagnosis of multiple myeloma, expresses questions that—so far as I can tell—virtually every person facing such a disease asks: "Why buy shoes? Why have dental work done?"[19] The plot of his story centers on desire: the narrative tension is whether lost desire will be regained. The initial loss of desire is expressed in indifference to such mundane acts as keeping up one's footwear and teeth. Diamond's story ends, happily, with him in a remission that is stable enough for him to want to buy shoes; he has made a transition from diagnostic shock to living with cancer. This plot of desire lost and regained informs all lives at various points, but illness demands reflection on cycles of when desire is lacking and when the body produces desire.

Just as illness almost invariably plunges the body into lacking desire, illness can instigate new reflections on how to be a body producing desire. Anatole Broyard describes critical illness as "like a great permission."[20] Part of what becomes permitted is the exploration of desires. Broyard writes that he began taking tap-dancing lessons after his diagnosis with prostate cancer. These lessons, besides probably being something he always wanted to do, were part of his self-conscious attempt "to develop a style" to meet his illness: "I think that only by insisting on your style can you keep from falling out of love with yourself as the illness attempts to diminish or disfigure you" (25).

Broyard's "falling out of love with yourself" gives life to my generic notion of "lacking desire," and "insisting on your style" says more than "producing desire" can capture. Yet generic terms are needed to point to what Broyard's language is doing and suggest relations between his sense of illness and that of others such as Diamond.

Broyard concludes that "it may not be dying we fear so much, but the diminished self" (25). What diminishes the self is no longer desiring for itself. Falling out of love with yourself means ceasing to consider yourself desirable to yourself: the ill person fears he is no longer worth clean teeth and new shoes.

As desire becomes reflective, an opening exists to assume enhanced responsibility for what is desired. Although desire is always for more than the immediate object—Diamond's shoes or Broyard's tap-dancing are self-consciously metonymic of a desire that will always exceed its tokens—the immediate objects remain ethical choices. For the dyadic body, productive desire leads to what Schweitzer called service.[21] Schweitzer's community of pain expresses a productive desire grounded in the ethical choice to be a body for other bodies.

Service can take many forms, but for the person who is seriously ill, a primary possibility for service is storytelling as an act of witness. As storytellers, writers like Broyard or Diamond do not tell people *how* to be sick; their testimony is rather that you *can* be sick and remain not just in love with yourself but in love with the humanity that shares sickness as its most fundamental commonality.

Four Ideal Typical Bodies

What are the four puppets that dance, and sometimes dangle, at the theoretical ends of these four continua? What are the types of action I invent in order to speak of the bodies in illness stories?

My typology of bodies is a meta-narrative, setting up different *choices* that body-selves then act out. The emphasis on choice is a reminder that the body is, ultimately, a moral problem, perhaps *the* moral problem a person has to address. Yet choice is also a deceptive word, because the body-self is created in reciprocal processes. Selves act in ways that choose their bodies, but bodies also create the selves who act. We can observe more of the first process than of the second; how bodies create selves is scarcely understood at all.

Matters are further complicated by noting that "choice" occurs in social contexts that constrain choice: conventions of stigma are one such constraint. But the post-colonial affirmations of stigma show that constraints on bodies can also become resources for body-selves. Broyard is constrained by the social undesirability of the body he is becoming, but he chooses to take tap-dancing lessons, as least as long as the flesh allows. He then turns tap-dancing into a story about the possibilities of choice.

People, particularly ill people, may not choose their bodies, but as body-selves they remain responsible for their bodies, and they choose how to exercise this responsibility. Those who observe others making choices have their own responsibility to note the conditions, both corporeal and social, that responsibility is exercised in.

The Disciplined Body

The disciplined body-self defines itself primarily in actions of *self-regimentation;* its most important action problems are those of control. The disciplined body experiences its gravest crisis in loss of control. The response of such a body-self is to reassert *predictability* through therapeutic regimens, which can be orthodox medical compliance or alternative treatment. In these regimens the body seeks to compensate for contingencies it cannot accept.

Such single-minded pursuit of regimens transforms the body into "it" to be treated; the self becomes *dissociated* from this "it." A self dissociated from its body will rarely seek and discover terms of association with others, so the disciplined body becomes *monadic.*

In its ideal-typical form the disciplined body *lacks* desire, and here real bodies most likely vary from the ideal type. The ideal type is most applicable in those moments of treatment when compliance becomes an end in itself. But few ill people pursue their regimens simply to demonstrate compliance to themselves or to their healers, without any desire for themselves. More often the pursuit of regimens indicates that something is desired; in Broyard's phrase, the body still loves itself. Often, but not always: Broyard offered this phrase because he recognized that many ill bodies cease to love themselves.

The disciplined body-self is not likely to tell stories about itself; rather, its stories are told through the pursuit of the regimen. Insofar as the regimen is the story, disciplined bodies can make "good patients" in terms of their medical compliance. Such a good patient is the medical equivalent of Robert Merton's ideal type, the ritualist, who has given up all hope of social success but continues to act out the prescribed norms of conduct.[22] Their demands are only in the cause of getting the regimen just right, and their expectations are surprisingly low, since performance of the regimen itself counts much more than its outcome.

The regimen need not be medical: diets, meditation programs, and exercise can complement or substitute for physicians' prescriptions. To the extent that these treatments are carried out like military drill, for the sole end of getting it right in itself, then desire is lacking and the pure ideal type is approximated. To the extent that the regimen provides pleasure—the food on the diet is preferred, the meditation or exercise are sources of relaxation and invigoration—then desire has become productive and something more than disciplined ritualism is being practiced.

Chemotherapy is perhaps the best example of the disciplined body's paradoxes of desire. Deborah Kahane narrates the story of a woman she interviewed, "Marcia." Marcia experiences breast cancer as a "tremendous relief." "I was finally being punished," she says, "and paying the price for being a bad mother and now it was over."[23] Other aspects of her story do not fit the monadic body, but in seeing cancer as a punishment, she is monadic in her self-isolation. Her phrase, "and now it was over," seems to refer to the period of awaiting a punishment she believes she deserves; if desire is present, it is masochistic.

Marcia also exemplifies the disciplined body as she works to restore predictability: she prides herself on returning to work soon after her mastectomy and on using a prosthesis to give her body a "normal" appearance. Then she suffers a recurrence and undergoes chemotherapy. Chemotherapy requires becoming a different sort of disciplined body: predictability becomes imposed, and body dissociation enters Marcia's story. "My whole life was planned around chemo treatments. I was wearing a wig and feeling lousy about my body" (123).

The tension that animates Marcia's story is whether she can move away from being a disciplined body, and she does. A crucial moment is her decision to end chemotherapy sooner than her physician advises. In that break from the prescribed regimen, she ceases to be a disciplined body. She makes peace with her aging body and finds new relationships as "a grandmother type" and a "mentor" (125). At the end of her story, far from interpreting cancer as a punishment, she now claims it as her own experience that has made her "more of a person for having survived" (127).

As a pure ideal type, the disciplined body is not a pleasant way to live. But most ill people experience some aspects of it: monadic self-enclosure, dissociation from a body that becomes "it," a need to restore some measure of control, and loss of desire. Marcia displays but never quite fits the ideal type of the disciplined body. Fortunately, she finally finds the terms to love herself.

The Mirroring Body

The mirroring body defines itself in acts of *consumption*. The body is both instrument and object of consuming: the body is used to consume, and consumption enhances the body: feeding it, clothing it, grooming it, and, in the consumption of medical services, curing it. This body-self is called mirroring because consumption attempts to recreate the body in the images of other bodies: more stylish and healthier bodies. The primary sense is visual: the body sees an image, idealizes it, and seeks to become the image of that image. The mirroring body thus attempts to make itself exactly what the popular phrase calls "the picture of health."

Like the disciplined body, the mirroring body seeks *predictability* because it fears contingency, but the kinds of contingency that the two bodies fear differ. The disciplined body typically fears contingencies that might disrupt work routines; it then substitutes health routines. The mirroring body fears disfigurement, which some disciplined bodies might regard as signs of battles well fought. Their respective attempts to ensure predictability will also differ. The disciplined body seeks predictability of performance; the mirroring body seeks predictability of appearance. If the disciplined body marches to the commands of an internalized drill sergeant, the mirroring body grooms itself in conformity to an internalized set of ideal images.

Both mirroring and disciplined bodies are also *monadic,* but again in differing ways. The disciplined body, set on its own course, regards others either as instrumental allies or obstacles. The mirroring body finds its course in the performance expectations of others who are its audience. Both bodies act alone in a world that judges them, but the judgments are made on different grounds: performance for the disciplined body and appearance for the mirroring body. Clearly many body-selves alternate between being disciplined bodies and mirroring bodies: Marcia alternates between speaking of her need to continue her work during illness and of the effect of illness on her appearance.

The mirroring body-self is almost compulsively *associated* with its body, but the body is now a surface; again, the visual is primary. The mirroring body *produces* desires, but its desire is monadic. What the mirroring body-self wants, it wants for itself.

If the disciplined body tells its story in its regimens, the mirroring body tells itself in its image, and this image comes from elsewhere. The images this body mirrors come most often from popular culture, where image is reality. Thus in one of the more bizarre new stories generated by Jacqueline Kennedy Onassis's death, Michael Jackson, whose book she had edited, was quoted expressing opposition to her having chemotherapy to treat non-Hodgkin's lymphoma: "She's too much of a legend to risk her hair falling out."[24] Whether Jackson said this or not, the tabloid writers have a clear enough sense of their readership to realize the statement would have sufficient popular resonance to make a story.

The reality of death is less real than the image of baldness. The identity of people who would take this story seriously is what Bauman described as "for today." What counts is sustaining the image today. As I have talked to people about to begin chemotherapy, a common reaction is for fears of immediate side-effects, particularly hair loss, to be more of a topic than fears of the treatment not working. Psychologists might call this a defense mechanism: the greater fear is displaced onto the lesser. But perhaps for some people whose identity truly is "for today," the immediate side-effects are the greater fear.[25]

Neither the Michael Jackson example nor its source are simply oddities. Tabloid journalism, advertisements, made-for-TV movies, and soap operas produce the images that most bodies seek to mirror. These images include both idealized health and pitiful illness; popular culture often plays one image against the other, idealizing health in contrast to illness, and depicting illness as pitiful in contrast to idealized health. Clearly other sources of images exist: families and medicine generate images of their own, though these images are often expressed in adaptations of popular culture. Professional culture is more "popular" than is imagined: prescription drug advertisements in medical trade magazines are presented in an iconography that is hard to distinguish from non-prescription ads in popular magazines.

The mirroring body does love itself, but this love is a parody of what Broyard probably meant; his point is that the body needs to be loved *with* the disfigurement brought by disease. As an ethical strategy for being ill—and each body type is an ethical strategy—the mirroring body has the same monadic limitations as the disciplined body. But consumer culture being as pervasive as sociology commonly proclaims, we are all mirroring bodies at one time or another.

Lacan's concept of the Imaginary suggests that what we call the self is always a sedimentation of images from elsewhere. These images are worn like armor, and what is within this armor is certainly less than we often believe. No self ever ceases living in the imaginary sedimentation of images from elsewhere. Thus, while the mirroring body has limited ethical possibilities, it remains as one inevitable facet of who most of us are. We can, however, complement our imaginary selves with entry into what Lacan calls the Symbolic. Here the body-self enters into symbolic exchanges: naming and being named are paradigmatic exchanges. Rather than simply appropriating others' images for itself, the body-self communicates with these others. Some exchanges with others are openings for ethical relationships; other exchanges, sadly, are not.

The Dominating Body

The dominating body defines itself in *force*. There is considerable cultural reluctance to talking about ill people, especially dying people, as being dominating bodies. Most people do not tell stories about themselves dominating others, and most certainly they do not write these stories down. Their narratives are lived, and the stories of these lives are told by others. Carole E. Andersen tells the story of the years her husband, Dick, was dying of leukemia.[26] Andersen observes that in the stories spouses tell about the death of a loved one, the dying person is invariably depicted as wise and courageous. "Bless them all," she writes, "their tales tell only one side of the story" (27).

As soon as he was diagnosed, Dick got mad. More precisely, he made anger into the narrative of his dying years, at least until the last months when his death was imminent and he did exhibit those qualities that surviving spouses idealize in their stories. But until those last months he was emotionally abusive in his possessiveness of Carole. The climax of this abuse came when he screamed her into the submissive act of giving up her part-time job writing a column in the local newspaper: "his words came as bullets; few of them missed. . . . He towered over me and let me have it—words, vile cruel words, repeated over and over again" (29). A psychologist she consults advises her to leave Dick, but she stays. Readers of her story can only hope that their last couple of months made the years worthwhile. Andersen's story is stark testimony to the reality of dominating bodies who are also ill.

The dominating body assumes the *contingency* of disease but never accepts it. Andersen tells that for twenty-seven months of the three-and-a-half years that Dick lived with leukemia, he was in remission, but it was the contingency of that remission, remission being defined as contingent, that drove him crazy. Dick "insisted he was afraid not of death but of the wait. It was never knowing that had haunted him" (31). Where the disciplined body turns its fear of contingency into the predictability of the regimen, the dominating body displaces rage against contingency onto other people. If Dick could not control his illness, he could control Carole.

The dominating body shares the qualities of *dissociation* and *lacking* desire with the disciplined body, with the crucial difference that the dominating body is *dyadic*. When the body is dissociated from itself but linked with others, the body's will turns against the other rather than toward itself. The aggression of this turning against others may reflect the bitterness of the dominating body's loss of desire. Andersen writes that at the time of his diagnosis, Dick loved life. But when his life was rendered contingent, he lost his desire. His bitterness comes from the knowledge that this *is* a loss. Contingency militates against desire throughout his illness. Even when he was in remission, Dick could no longer take pleasure in the life he had so enjoyed. Finally when his death was certain and "once again he felt in control," Dick became the husband Carole loved.

Although the dominating body is dyadic in its other-relatedness, the ethical stance of this dyadic relation is *against* others rather than *for* others. Being dyadic toward others while dissociated from itself, and while lacking desire, is dangerous. The disciplined and mirroring bodies turn on themselves. The dominating body turns on others. Society does not want to hear the resulting narrative of abusive force, but as Carole Andersen puts it, if both those dying within this narrative and their loved ones are to be helped, "then it's time for some honesty" (28).

The Communicative Body

The disciplined, mirroring, and dominating bodies are ideal types; no actual body fits their specifications, at least for long,[27] but these specifications provide some interpretive understanding of how bodies exist at different moments of their being. The communicative body-self is not only an ideal type but also an *idealized* type. Its specifications are not only descriptive but provide an ethical ideal for bodies. Again, no actual body fits this ideal for long, though many bodies may approximate it in differing ways.[28]

The communicative body accepts its *contingency* as part of

the fundamental contingency of life. The human body, for all its resilience, is fragile; breakdown is built into it. Bodily predictability, if not the exception, should be regarded as exceptional; contingency ought to be accepted as normative. The communicative body-self takes its place in Schweitzer's "brotherhood of those who bear the mark of pain."

This contingent body is fully *associated* with itself. The communicative body understands that the body-self exists as a unity, with its two parts not only interdependent but inextricable. There may be aspects of body that are not self, and *vice versa,* but just where one ends and the other begins is undecidable. Thus no distinction between corporeal disease and illness experience can be sustained: a problem within the tissues pervades the whole life.

Association and contingency are contextualized by the qualities of *being dyadic* and *producing desire,* and these qualities crystallize the body's ethical dimension. When a body that associates with its own contingency turns outward in dyadic relatedness, it sees reflections of its own suffering in the bodies of others. When the body is a desiring one, the person wants and needs to relieve the suffering of others. Here lies the sense of obligation toward the other that grounds Schweitzer's "brotherhood of those who bear the mark of pain": the dyadic desire of the communicative body means that it never belongs to itself alone but constructs its humanity in relation to other bodies.

The communicative body realizes the ethical ideal of existing *for* the other. The *communing body* might be more precise, but I retain "communicative" as the more general term. The communion of bodies involves a communication of recognition that transcends the verbal. Bodies commune in touch, in tone, in facial expression and gestural attitude, and in breath. Communication is less a matter of content than of *alignment:* when bodies sense themselves in alignment with others, words make sense in the context of that alignment. When alignment is lacking, even the best semantic content risks misinterpretation or will be unsatisfactory as a message.

The body itself *is* the message; humans commune through their bodies. Anatole Broyard wrote that he wanted "to be a good story" for his physician.[29] The phrase catches the reader off guard; conventionally, the ill person would say something like "I want him to listen to my story." Broyard incites the recognition that his ill body *is* a story, and he wants it to be a good one. The remark occurs as Broyard talks about the ill person's need to personify his illness and to "own" it, rather than allow it to be the anonymous disease that medicine depicts. Ethics seems to begin in a similar sense of ownership of situations; responsibility as an ethical person involves making a good story of the situation that self and other find themselves in and must come to own.

Like the disciplined, mirroring, and dominating bodies, the communicative body *is* a story, but a wholly different one. The communicative body *communes* its story with others; the story invites others to recognize themselves in it. Thus the communicative body tells itself explicitly in stories. Reciprocally, stories are the medium of bodies seeking to approximate the communicative type.

Human communication with the world, and the communion this communication rests on, begins in the body. "I can understand the nature of the living being outside of myself," Schweitzer wrote, "only through the living being within me."[30] This statement is an essential epigram of the communicative body-self, with its confluence of *associated* body-relatedness and *dyadic* other-relatedness. Schweitzer's joint emphases on suffering as life's inevitable *contingency* and on service as a *productive* desire to join with other bodies express the full ethical ideal of the communicative body.

        o   o   o

In the diagram that orients this chapter, the flat linearity of type and the constraint of matrix space renders matters too neat. I reiterate several points about this false appearance of neatness to emphasize the four ideal types only present rough parameters for the action choices of body-selves.

For each range of responses to action problems, the paired terms—such as predictable/contingent in relation to the problem of control—mark the ends of a continuum. Thus in the really real, bodies act not at the extremes but anywhere along these continua. Moreover, the quality of each extreme can change: thus body association can be naive to suffering or accepting of it, and contingency can be feared or embraced.

How far along the body is placed on any continuum sometimes represents embracing that condition, as the communicative body embraces being dyadic. The body's placement can also represent a resistance to the opposite end of that continuum: the disciplined body makes itself predictable as resistance to its fundamental contingency, and the dominating body lacks desire because its contingency seems to deny what it desires to desire. The "continua" thus have a shape that defies conventional geometrical metaphors, as well as two-dimensional printing.

Clearly then the four body types cannot be either mutually exclusive or exhaustive. Other permutations certainly have descriptive force, and because the body is moving in time, the condition of any actual body represents a layering of types. Each of us is not one type or another, but a shifting foreground and background of types. The value of the types is to describe the extreme moments of these shifts, thus providing some parameters for hearing the body in the story.

Finally, because my objective is an ethics of the body, I am mixing three ideal types with one *idealized* type. My typology seeks to be normative not in a descriptive sense but in a prescriptive one. I want to show how the communicative body distinguishes itself from other body types. By specifying the communicative body as the undertaking of an ethical task, I hope to orient an ethics of the body. Reflexive monitoring requires an ideal against which the progress of the body-self can be measured.

The next chapter turns to stories, to their role in illness and their context in postmodern times. Chapters 4 through 6 propose three basic illness narratives which most actual stories exemplify. These narratives are not presented as linguistic structures, but as objectifications of the bodies that tell them. The narratives are shown to be media for body-selves to express and reflexively monitor themselves.

My thesis is that different bodies have "elective affinities" to different illness narratives. These elective affinities are not deterministic. Bodies are realized—not just represented but created—in the stories they tell. This realization can and should be reflexive: by telling certain stories, ethical choices are made; the choices in turn generate stories. Common sense understands people as having some responsibility for their stories and for their bodies. Common sense is less accustomed to the possibility of exercising that responsibility for bodies *through* stories.

One road to the achievement of the communicative body is through storytelling. The final chapters, on testimony and ethics, develop the communicative body as an ethical ideal for living with illness.

Three

Three

*Illness as a Call
for Stories*

"We are forever telling stories about ourselves," writes the psychoanalyst Roy Schafer.[1] Schafer's work is seminal in understanding how selves are perpetually recreated in stories. Stories do not simply describe the self; they are the self's medium of being. Where the last chapter emphasized the body part of the body-self, this chapter emphasizes the self. In particular, it considers selves and stories from the perspective of illness: how is illness an occasion for stories; what needs do the ill address in their stories? The chapter concludes by inquiring into the affinity between illness stories and postmodern times.

Narrative Wreckage

Becoming seriously ill is a call for stories in at least two senses.[2] The first is what Judith Zaruches implies when she writes of losing her map and destination. Stories have to *repair* the damage that illness has done to the ill person's sense of where she is in life, and where she may be going. Stories are a way of redrawing maps and finding new destinations.

The second and complementary call for stories is literal and immediate: the phone rings and people want to know what is happening to the ill person. Stories of the illness have to be told to medical workers, health bureaucrats, employers and work

redraw maps

all that happened

associates, family and friends. Whether ill people want to tell stories or not, illness calls for stories.

The spring when I was writing this book I had a routine chest X-ray that showed enlarged lymph nodes; the chest is the expected recurrence site for the cancer I had. The inflammation turned out not to be cancer, but in the course of medical tests and finally surgery, I had to tell and repeat versions of my story to family with their interests, work colleagues with theirs, and to medical workers who required still different stories. One day I recorded I had told a version of my illness story eight times.

These stories are told in conditions of fatigue, uncertainty, sometimes pain, and always fear that turn the ill person into what Ronald Dworkin describes as a "narrative wreck," a phrase displaying equal wit and empathy.[3] Judith Zaruches's metaphor of losing her map and destination suggests illness as a shipwreck. Almost every illness story I have read carries some sense of being shipwrecked by the storm of disease, and many use this metaphor explicitly. Extending this metaphor describes storytelling as repair work on the wreck.

The repair begins by taking stock of what survives the storm. The old map may now be less than useful, but it has hardly been carbonized. Disease happens in a life that already has a story, and this story goes on, changed by illness but also affecting how the illness story is formed. I once spoke to a young man the night before he began chemotherapy. He talked about the high incidence of cancer in his family, his father's recent death, and his memories of relatives' deaths. At least on that particular night as he recalled his life, he told a story of having waited for cancer; a story of illness was already in place before his disease occurred. Cancer had long been on his map as a possible destination.

Yet he was a narrative wreck for at least two reasons. However cancer may be anticipated in fantasy, the reality is different. When I was told about the lymph nodes on my chest X-ray, I was amazed at what a narrative wreck I was: I who spend my life telling stories about illness, my own as well as others. Somehow the stories we have in place never fit the reality, and sometimes this disjunction can be worse than having no story at all.

My friend was also a narrative wreck because he, like anyone facing serious illness, had suddenly lost the central resource that any storyteller depends on: a sense of temporality. The conventional expectation of any narrative, held alike by listeners and storytellers, is for a past that leads into a present that sets in place a foreseeable future. The illness story is wrecked because its present is not what the past was supposed to lead up to, and the future is scarcely thinkable.

Recall Malcolm Diamond's questions about whether he should have dental work done or buy shoes. These questions are not only about desire but about temporality: Diamond has lost any stable expectation of a relation between what he does in the present and what will happen in the future. Even if death is not an immediate concern, what tomorrow may have in store for the body is unknown. At least I can make known what happened to the young man with so much cancer in his family: the chemotherapy was successful, and in remission he is moving to new destinations.

The way out of the narrative wreckage is telling stories, specifically those stories that Schafer calls "self-stories." The self-story is not told for the sake of description, though description may be its ostensible content. The self is being *formed* in what is told. The quotation from Schafer that began this chapter continues: "In telling these self-stories *to others* we may, for most purposes, be said to be performing straightforward narrative actions. In saying that we also tell them *to ourselves*, however, we are enclosing one story within another. This is the story that there is a self to tell something to, a someone else serving as audience who is oneself or one's self. . . . On this view, the self is a telling."[4]

The self-story is told both to others and to one's self; each telling is enfolded within the other. The act of telling is a dual reaffirmation. Relationships with others are reaffirmed, and the self is reaffirmed. Serious illness requires both reaffirmations, and Schafer's insight is describing how they proceed mutually. The ill person needs to reaffirm that his story is worth listening to by others. He must also reaffirm that *he is still there*, as an audience for himself. Audre Lorde's expression of her need to write after her surgery for breast cancer begins, "In order to keep me available to myself. . . ."[5] Illness is a crisis of self in the specific sense of an uncertainty that one's self is still there as an audience; the reaffirmation of this self as "available" is crucial.

No pretense can be made of reviewing the massive literature bearing on Schafer's thesis that "the self is a telling."[6] But I can suggest certain themes from this literature that seem most pertinent to hearing illness stories.

INTERRUPTION AND PURPOSE

In the beginning is an interruption. Disease interrupts a life, and illness then means living with perpetual interruption.[7] Nancy Mairs writes that calamities "have a genius of their own."[8] Mairs's life has been interrupted by her own mental and physical illnesses and her husband's recurring cancer, by children and their needs, and by the needs of strangers and her sense of obligation to meet those needs. Finally, as her self-story is about to reconcile belief in God with the indignities of having multiple sclerosis, she writes that "the lid just popped off my daily Thirstbuster, dumping about a quart of Diet Coke onto the floor." Mairs is too disabled to clean up the mess and will "have to continue working on this passage with my feet in a sticky brown puddle" (184).

Mairs interrupts her story in order to display the constant interruption of her life. Her story not only describes these interruptions; it is an interrupted story. The passage also illustrates how metaphor often works in illness stories. The spill is a metaphor for Mairs's interrupted life, but the sticky brown puddle is literal. Thus with regard to metaphor I find most useful Schafer's observation that metaphor establishes a storyline: "What is called unpacking a metaphor is in certain respects much like laying out the kinds of story that are entailed by the metaphor." Between storyline and metaphor, Schafer finds the former to be "the more inclusive term."[9]

The lid popping off interrupts one storyline in order to establish another. The digression is a reminder that her story is about interruption, or, in Schafer's terms, interruption is the story entailed by the metaphor. Mairs's body is equally entailed: her story is a body-self-story. The popped lid jerks the reader back into awareness of the physical conditions that are both the topic of Mairs's writing and the means of performing that writing. Her metaphor is her story of what it is like to live in a body so disabled that she can only sit in the sticky brown puddle until help arrives. She is not helpless: her work can continue. But the condition of that work's embodiment is perpetual vulnerability to interruption.

The Thirstbuster lid may have had a genius of its own, but other interruptions are explicitly part of the territory of being ill. The ill person as medical patient is one who, having been interrupted by disease, is now considered infinitely interruptible in speech, schedule, sleep, solvency, and anything else. When Richard Selzer, writing of his recovery from a coma caused by Legionnaires' disease, is asked by his physician why he wants to be discharged from the hospital, Selzer replies that he wants not just privacy—he already has a private room; he wants "solitude. A condition that does not include people like you coming in here whenever they feel like it and asking me what else I want."[10] Even the most benevolent interruption remains an intrusion when it is uninvited. Selzer's irony suggests that he interprets the interruptions to be benevolent; others may not share this understanding.

The medical redefinition of conversation between physician and patient as a clinical task, for example, as "history taking," works to suspend normal conventions of politeness and thus to legitimate interruptions. Physicians' interruptions of patients are well-documented.[11] The physician and sociologist Howard Waitzkin interprets these interruptions as "basically attempts to curtail storytelling by patients." Waitzkin suggests several reasons for this curtailment: "The story may not contribute to the doctor's cognitive process of reaching a diagnosis; the patient's version of the story may be confusing or inconsistent; telling the story may take more time than is perceived to be available; or parts of the story may create feelings that are uncomfortable for the doctor, the patient, or both."[12] Times are changing. A senior surgeon wrote to me that he is finally learning the difference between taking a history and hearing the patient's story; until recently, the medical history was considered to be the story.

Telling an interrupted life requires a new kind of narrative. Mairs cuts to the inconsistency between interruption and conventional storytelling: "Narratives possess the shortcoming that they drive toward ends, preferably tidy ones."[13] Interruptions divert the narrative from such ends; they give stories the "confusing or inconsistent" quality that Waitzkin observes physicians and patients find uncomfortable in patients' stories. The stories are uncomfortable, and their uncomfortable quality is all the more reason they have to be told. Otherwise, the interrupted voice remains silenced.

The illness story faces a dual task. The narrative attempts to restore an order that the interruption fragmented, but it must also tell the truth that interruptions will continue. Part of this truth is that the tidy ends are no longer appropriate to the story. A different kind of end—a different purpose—has to be discovered. The result is rarely tidy: "Even as I write about it," concludes Fitzhugh Mullan on his cancer, "I can feel a kind of terminal ambivalence about the entire experience."[14] Many illness stories do discover purposes in suffering, but even these are rarely without some ambivalence.

Interrupted narratives find many different purposes, and these will be considered in the following chapters. The most general terms of purpose are suggested by Genevieve Lloyd, describing Nietzsche's concept of the eternal return: "It is a matter rather of seeing everything that happens—whether it be grand or unbearably petty—as integral to the being of a self which, if it were to recur at all, could do so only in its entirety."[15] Nancy Mairs interrupts her meditations on God to describe the Thirstbuster spilling: the lesson of her interruption is that the grand is never far from the petty.

MEMORY AND RESPONSIBILITY

The interruption that illness is, and the further interruptions that it brings, are disruptions of memory. The disruption is not of remembering; people's memories of illness are often remarkable in their precision and duration. I was once on a radio phone-in program. A man called and told a detailed story of having cancer; his wife was hospitalized at the same time that he was, and the details of their visits went on at a length that made the program host nervous. I finally asked the man when this had happened and was told it was thirty years ago. I am frequently amazed at how long ago "present tense" stories have happened. The disturbance is not of remembering, but it is of memory.

The memory that is disrupted is a coherent sense of life's sequence: what the philosopher David Carr calls "the whole which comprises future, present, and past."[16] I suggested above how illness dislocates the relation of this whole: the present is not what the past was supposed to lead to, and whatever future will follow this present is contingent. Carr points out that even for the healthy person, "the narrative coherence of events and actions" is never "simply a 'given' for us. Rather it is a constant task, sometimes a *struggle,* and when it succeeds it is an achievement" (96, emphasis added).

Illness intensifies that struggle. The past is remembered with such arresting lucidity because it is not being experienced as past; the illness experiences that are being told are unassimilated fragments that refuse to become past, haunting the present. Just as present illness struggles with a past that was not supposed to lead to illness, the present that is recovered from illness struggles with a past that never received its due telling when it was happening.

Disrupted memory—whatever the incoherence in the whole which comprises future, present, and past—is a *moral* problem. Developing arguments from Alasdair MacIntyre, Carr describes this struggle as "a responsibility which no one else can finally lift entirely from the shoulders of the one who lives that life." This struggle has two aspects: "one to live out or live up to a plan or narrative, large or small, particular or general; the other to construct or choose that narrative. The first is constrained by the choice of the second" (96). For the ill, the choice of narrative is equally constrained by a sense of what can be lived out or, in Carr's significant phrase, *lived up to.*

The practical problem of narrative, according to Carr, is to create a story in which "the past is still viewed in light of its connection to present and future in an ongoing project" (98). In such a narrative, memory is restored as coherent. Because the present of illness is not what was planned in the past, reestablishing the connection of past to present may require an exercise in what psychoanalyst Donald Spence calls narrative truth. Spence and Carr agree that the past cannot be reinvented, but the sense of what was foreground and background in past events can shift to recreate a past that displays what Spence calls greater "continuity and closure."[17] Out of narrative truths a sense of coherence can be restored.

Even the ill person can choose a narrative and create narrative truths. The story expressing these truths must then be *told*. Psychologist Roger Schank is clearest on the need to tell stories to others, although actual telling is implicit in the writing of Schafer and Spence, who both assume psychoanalysis as the scene of storytelling. Schank explicitly links telling to memory: "We need to tell someone else a story that describes our experience because the process of creating a story also *creates the memory structure* that will contain the gist of the story for the rest of our lives. Talking is remembering."[18] Memory is not only restored in the illness story; more significantly, memory is created. If the story being told is what Carr calls something to live up to, then a future is also being created, and that future carries a distinct responsibility.

Paul Ricoeur makes this responsibility central to his concept of *narrative identity*. Ricoeur describes how the self only comes to be in the process of the life story being told: "the *subject* is never given at the beginning" of a narrative. This initial non-givenness of the subject or self is a necessary condition of the story's morality. If the subject were given at the beginning, nothing would be learned. Such an already-given subject would, in Ricoeur's phrase, "run the risk of reducing itself to a narcissistic ego, self-centered and avaricious." Narrative identity is the liberation from this narcissism of being a narrator who believes he already knows who he is. "In place of an ego enchanted by itself a *self* is born" in stories.[19]

This responsibility for narrative identity is directly expressed in illness stories. Tim Brookes, writing about his life with asthma, comes to the realization that "chronic illness in particular challenges us to ask if it is possible to be *successfully ill.*"[20] The ethicist William May reflects on the response of a recent widow to her husband's sudden death. The question faced by the ill person is not "What are we going to do about it?" May observes; rather, it is "How does one rise to the occasion?"[21]

Briefly, one rises to the occasion by telling not just any story, but a good story. This good story is the measure of an ill person's success. "Narrative truth is what we have in mind when we say that such and such is a good story," Spence writes.[22] In chapter 2, I quoted Anatole Broyard describing himself as wanting to be a "good story" for his doctor.

Broyard said this during a speech to doctors; in that context, he is proposing a mutuality of responsibility that is new both to illness experience and to medicine. Broyard claims a role far beyond that of compliant patient. His responsibility is not that defined by Parsons for the sick person, to get well by following medical advice. Instead Broyard claims a responsibility to turn his illness into a good story, to discover the narrative truth in it, and to tell that truth. He is declaring himself a witness to his illness, and he is calling on his audience—members of the medical profession—to become witnesses to his witness. Broyard knew without reading Schank that a story requires listeners; it must be told. As he assumed responsibility for being a good story, he called on his physicians to take the complementary responsibility for receiving this story.

The narrative truth of the good story has to remain truthful to life as it is lived; the question is, which truth of which happenings? In illness stories, truth may be selective, but it remains self-conscious. This accountability of truth is close to the surface of illness stories. One day I met a friend whose adult child is mentally disabled; she was just back from a parents' support group. "We do not tell our own truth," she said to me, describing the group. These parents, my friend told me, were unwilling to tell their disappointments and frustrations. The raw anguish of such talk was rendered unacceptable by unspoken group norms. But telling the truth, as my friend knew, involves recognizing that your life has not turned out as you wanted. What went wrong must be acknowledged and examined; mourning will attend this examination.

Many if not most North Americans share a cultural reluctance to say that their lives have gone badly in some significant respect and to mourn the loss of what was desired but will never happen. Our contemporary version of stoicism borders on denial. The good story refuses denial, and thus stands against social pressures. Waitzkin points out that physicians interrupt patients when their stories become uncomfortable. The interruptions work to silence the telling of what might be, or what might become, truths. What might have become good stories are turned; if not turned bad, then at least turned away from their truths.

What makes an illness story good is the act of witness that says, implicitly or explicitly, "I will tell you not what you want to hear but what I know to be true because I have lived it. This truth will trouble you, but in the end, you cannot be free without it, because you know it already; your body knows it already." In telling this story truthfully, the ill person rises to the occasion.

More needs to be said about the ill person as witness, and a later chapter will return to this theme. Here I only observe that the possibility of becoming a witness makes the coherence of memory the responsibility that Carr calls it. Memory is a responsibility because as it is told it becomes witness and reaches

beyond the individual into the consciousness of the community.

RECLAIMING THE SELF

In postmodern times "reclaiming" has been used to the point of cliché, but like most clichés it carries a significant kernel of truth about the times in which it is so often repeated. Reclaiming suggests that illness stories are doing more than speaking through interruptions; the ill person's voice has been taken away.

Audre Lorde writes of "reclaiming . . . that language which has been made to work against us."[23] She expresses a pervasive view among the ill that medical language with its "general unifying view" homogenizes their experience. Students of medical culture find "doctor stories" to be rich in their descriptive nuance,[24] but the issue is whether patients experience this side of medicine. Too often the patient experiences a medical rationalization that is epitomized by "diagnostic related groups" (DRGs).

DRGs are detailed statements of what medical treatments some third party insurer will pay for, based on the diagnosis at the time of hospital admission. The DRG is a narrative that sets in place details of the experience of the hospitalization that will follow. I was going to write "countless details," but the logic of the DRG is that every detail, down to the last paper tissue, can and will be counted. The DRG reduces the general unifying view to bureaucratic proceduralism. Again, to characterize medical narrative culture in terms of DRGs is certainly unfair, but DRGs do epitomize the dehumanizing aspect of "becoming a patient" described by Dan Gottlieb in chapter 1.

The finest statement of the practice of reclaiming is by Audre Lorde: "In order to keep me available to myself, and be able to concentrate my energies upon the challenges of those worlds through which I move, I must consider what my body means to me."[25] To reclaim a self requires making the self available as what Schafer called an audience to its own self-story. But Lorde's story, like Mairs's, is a body-self-story. Her reclaiming begins with her body: the problem of how to regain association with her body after her mastectomy. Her need for self-availability, however, goes beyond her body-self. To be available to herself as a one-breasted woman, she must find a connection to all who share that condition. How the medical world she moves through challenges this connection is described in a later chapter. Lorde must reclaim herself against this opposition.

Lorde echoes William James's call to the "duties" of the really real. The reclaiming that begins in her body moves seamlessly to the "challenges of those worlds" she moves through. She reminds the ill, and herself, that the worlds any of us move through are challenging, and illness requires an enhanced concentration of energies to meet those challenges. This concentration requires, and in another sense *is*, what Lorde calls self-availability. She makes herself available to herself in the words the reader reads. Her writing is her struggle for coherence; its truth is her achievement. Not just any story will bring about this coherence. Lorde's good story is one that concentrates her energies and returns her to the worlds that need her. Lorde's reader is simultaneously reminded of her own worlds and their challenges; thus the reader is made available to herself.

Lorde's telling is an act of reflexive monitoring. As narrative practice, reflexivity is described by Jerome Bruner in terms of restoring memory: "our capacity to turn around on the past and alter the present in its light, or to alter the past in the light of the present."[26] Reflexive monitoring is the perpetual readjustment of past and present to create and sustain a good story. Lorde's narrative practice is exactly what Schafer, Carr, Spence, and Schank all call for: the creation of a coherent self-story, the re-creation of memory, and the assumption of responsibility. But Lorde emphasizes what none of these theorists include: by calling her narrative work a reclaiming, she attends to its political dimension.

What Lorde believes she must reclaim is suggested by returning to Waitzkin's analysis of doctor-patient communications. Waitzkin characterizes medicine as an ideological system that "calls" the patient to be an identity that medicine maintains for him; the diagnosis is the most prevalent form of this identity. The ideological work of medicine is to get the patient to accept this diagnostic identity as appropriate and moral.[27] When the patient accepts this identity, he aligns himself as subordinate in a power relation. Parsons's frequent emphasis on the asymmetry of the professional-client relationship remains forceful because it legitimizes this power relation, endowing it with a certain inevitability. Waitzkin recognizes that for the patient, "the language of medicine leaves few options for action. . . . Periodically, such tensions that derive from troubling social issues erupt into the discourse . . . and create a countertextual reality that cannot be resolved in the framework of a medical encounter" (47). Lorde's reclaiming is such a countertextual reality.

Few illness stories are as self-consciously political as Audre Lorde's, but few are without some motivation of reclaiming. Her statement about self-availability is as good an epigram as I have found to the narrative practice of illness stories, but one significant addition must be made. Just as Lorde specifies the plurality of the worlds she moves through, so also the plurality of the self that is reclaimed needs to be noted. The issue for most ill people seems to be keeping multiple selves available to themselves. Stewart Alsop observes that his book "was written by different mes."[28]

Alsop's self-observation confirms the generalized significance of what Schafer notes among analysands: the "experiential self may be seen as a set of varied narratives that seem to be told by and about a cast of varied selves. And yet, like the dream, the entire tale is told by one narrator. Nothing here supports the common illusion that there is a single self-entity that each person has and experiences, a self-entity that is, so to speak, out there in Nature."[29] What is out there in Nature is, of course, the body. There may be a cast of varied selves, but there seems to be only one body; how many selves can this one body support?

Two sorts of answers are posed by different stories. Sue Nathanson writes about the years following the traumas of an abortion and a tubal ligation. These were elective procedures, fully understood and consented to, and no distinctive medical horrors occurred. But Nathanson could not anticipate how much losing her baby and her fertility would mean to her. She repeatedly tells her readers that her energies had been primarily focused not on her career as a professional psychotherapist but on child bearing and nurturing. Foreclosing that part of her life is a trauma that takes years to resolve.

Part of the resolution is Nathanson's realization that she is not one person but many, and some parts of her have to act in ways that contradict the values of other parts. As she counsels a young woman who has had an abortion, Nathanson articulates her own developing self-awareness: "Women have to . . . accept the consciousness of having the power and capacity to end a life that is also part of their very being," she says.[30] Nathanson realizes that her own cast of varied selves includes the destroyer and the nurturer, and these selves can co-exist. The work of telling her self-story is a process of getting rid of what Schafer calls the "exaggerated impression of single and unvarying self-entities."[31]

A different and equally dramatic resolution to the problem of a single body supporting varied selves is found in Reynolds Price's story of surgery, radiation, and recovery from a malignant tumor within his spinal column. Price describes in detail how the paralysis that results from radiation affects his life. His conclusion is that he now inhabits a body that is fundamentally different, and thus he must be a different person. He advises any who suffer similar fates to become "someone else, the next viable you—a stripped-down whole and clear-eyed person, realistic as a sawed-off shotgun and thankful for air."[32] A new body calls for a new self, nothing less will do. Others, especially those who love the ill person most, "will be hard at work in the fierce endeavor to revive your old self, the self they recall with love and respect" (183). Their benevolent efforts must be resisted.

How "new" Price's self-proclaimed new self is can be disputed, but the narrative truth of his story is clear: in thinking of himself as a new self, he has found the terms to go on living in conditions of embodiment that would have horrified his old self. And he witnesses to others the possibility of creating a "*happy*" life out of such circumstances (192).

What unites the narrative reclaimings of Lorde, Nathanson, and Price is summarized by Lloyd, writing about the primal teller of self-stories, Augustine. "Reflection on memory makes the self an object of wonder—an astonishment previously reserved for the contemplation of the world."[33] The good story ends in wonder, and the capacity for wonder is reclaimed from the bureaucratic rationalizations of institutional medicine. Being available to yourself ultimately means having the ability to wonder at all the self can be.

NARRATIVE WRECKAGE AND POSTMODERN TIMES

Illness is one specific occasion for narrative wreckage, but a condition of perpetual narrative uncertainty is endemic to postmodern times. The self-stories that proliferate in postmodern times are one response to this uncertainty. This proliferation of self-stories includes the analytic self-stories that Schafer refers to and the self-stories that the ill tell from their bedsides. But far more widespread are self-stories as a recognizable genre of popular culture.

Illness narratives as one form of self-story overlap with and are bounded by at least three other forms. These are spiritual autobiographies,[34] stories of becoming a man or a woman and what that gender identity involves,[35] and finally survivor stories of inflicted traumas such as war, captivity, incest, and abuse.[36] As in illness stories, the published examples of these self-stories are only a token of a broader oral discourse. The ways that oral stories are influenced by the rhetoric of published works are undoubtedly as infinite as those stories.

Why is this proliferation of self-stories happening *now*? In terms of published stories, one answer is that a market exists, and this market in turn means readers who find this storytelling addresses their lives. Published self-stories are another ideology, though disputedly a more grass-roots one, that "calls" people to the identities it formulates. But the presence of this market only enlarges the scope of the question, why now?

Each of these self-stories is grounded in some form of narrative wreckage, and each is its own act of reclaiming. Postmodern times both produces the wreckage and provides the resources for the reclaiming. Postmodernity is, in this as in most other respects, contradictory: opposing tendencies happen simultaneously. One side of postmodernity is the hyper-rationalization that subsumes the individuality extolled by modernity. Modernist medicine's general unifying view was a beneficent rationalization carried out in the interest of a science that had cure as its objective. DRGs are a less-than-beneficent rationalization carried out in the interest of cost-containment and administrative control over medicine. DRGs represent the modernist project turning against itself.

A different side of postmodernity is the presence of self-stories that provide models of reclaiming the self. To see this side, the practitioners of postmodernism are more useful than theorists, though another feature of postmodernism is the blurring of this line. One practitioner is the novelist Clark Blaise. In the preface to his own self-story, Blaise defines the narrative implications of postmodern times as "consciousness fighting to achieve sovereignty over its own experience."[37] Blaise echoes but intensifies Schafer's observation that experience is "made or fashioned" and not directly encountered, as well as Carr's recognition that coherence is always a struggle. He also echoes John Lennon's reported saying, "Reality takes a lot of imagination." In postmodern times William James's really real is still there, but where it is and what it is require more work. To experience we have to imagine; imagination is consciousness struggling to gain sovereignty over its experience.

The modernist autobiographer—still represented by politicians and other "personalities"—presents his story's ending, the culmination of the status that the author has achieved, as somehow immanent in the story throughout. The postmodern memoirist like Blaise is haunted by the mutual contingency of life and story. Because imagination knows that the story could always be told differently, should the life have been lived differently?

The postmodern memoirist writes to discover what other selves were operating, unseen, in a story that is the writer's own, but that writer is several selves. As Nathanson tells her story, she is a *writer* telling how she as a *therapist* spoke to her client about what she as a *woman* who had suffered learned about the *multiple sides* of herself. The story she tells the other person, her client, is also a story she is telling herself, thus creating a new memory, possibly for both of them. Here we certainly have Schafer's cast of varied selves.

The anything-but-tidy conventions of postmodern memoir

—its lack of linearity and competing voices—fit experiences that are interrupted. As I observed earlier, these stories are not only about interruption; they are themselves interrupted stories. Not the least interruption are other stories. Another storyteller, the therapist, group leader, and spiritual autobiographer Sam Keen begins with the commonplace observation that in postmodern times people can no longer participate in some shared communal belief(s) about matters such as "soul" and "guiding principles."[38] The storyteller's perception that Keen brings to this observation is that in a world without these principles, the narrator becomes "saturated with stories . . . with points of view." A person who is "bombarded" with so many points of view has to struggle to hold one point of view that can be recognized as her own. The unique perspective that makes the story one's own constantly breaks up in competing perspectives. "We lose the continuity of our experiences," Keen writes; "we become people who are written on from the outside" (28).

When I had to repeat the story of the X-ray that led to suspected cancer, I began to feel after multiple tellings that a voice outside of me was talking, and I was listening to that voice. I was not speaking of how *I* felt; I was addressing the interests of particular listeners in rhetoric appropriate to our relationships. I felt written on from the outside, but my own voice was doing the writing.

The postmodern phrase that complements "reclaiming" is "finding one's voice." Here also a significant truth underpins the cliché: people who are written on from the outside have lost their voices. Speaking in a voice recognizable as one's own becomes increasingly difficult, so speech proliferates in search of that voice. Self-stories proliferate.

Amid the cast of various selves, which self can speak the voice that is one's "own"? The question is not facetious, because the need to speak in a voice recognizable as one's own is real. The best answer I have found is offered by Nancy Mairs, reflecting on the question she is always asked when she visits undergraduate writing classes, "How did you find your voice?"[39] After some discussion of the invented quality of any voice, Mairs writes: "Whatever I wrote, I wrote out of that pain, and whatever I wrote assuaged the pain a little but never enough" (19). Even in postmodern times, even among the various selves that each of us is, a bedrock of the really real remains. Its name is often pain.

Again I ask, why do self-stories proliferate now? Perhaps because the accumulated violences of modernity are no longer deniable, which is another definition of postmodernity. Terry Tempest Williams tells a story of breast cancer, not her own but throughout her family.[40] Because so many women are affected in a fairly short period of time, she seeks some environmental cause. Part of any story of illness is genesis: what caused the disease; why did it happen to me?[41] But in Williams's case the question is why cancer is happening all around her.

Near the end of her book Williams tells her father about her recurring dream of a bright light. He tells her this is actually a memory of the family stopping their car by the Utah roadside to watch an atomic bomb test in the 1950s. "The sky seemed to vibrate with an eerie pink glow," he tells her. "Within a few minutes, a light ash was raining on the car." She stares at him as the question of genesis suddenly becomes clear: "It was at this moment that I realized the deceit I had been living under" (283).

The "deceit" is more complicated than atomic testing. It involves her family's Mormon tradition of authority, their relation to the Western landscape, and the "unnatural history" of that landscape, particularly the Great Salt Lake region. When all these complications have been explored, a final mystery of genesis remains: why, among all the women who suffered from the fallout of that and other explosions, does Williams alone survive?

Williams tells a self-story of memory and responsibility. Her story is multiply interrupted, by floods, deaths, and ultimately by her father's revelation that is not exactly the truth but is at least the end of a denial. Whatever "finding your own voice" means, in ending the denial Williams certainly finds a purpose for her voice: honoring her dead and struggling to preserve the natural heritage that is being destroyed by forces as insidious as that bomb was.

The postmodernism of her story lies in all these qualities, as well as in the anachronism of the atomic testing that seems part of another world, yet has such real effects here and now. "When the Atomic Energy Commission described the country north of the Nevada Test Site as 'virtually uninhabited desert terrain,'" Williams writes, "my family and the birds at Great Salt Lake were some of the 'virtual uninhabitants'" (287). Here the practices of modernity create the language of postmodernism.[42]

In terms of total pages, most of Williams's book is not about illness but about nature; she is a bird watcher by choice and turns to illness only when its interruption demands response. She struggles for the sovereignty of her consciousness over the events of her life, and she struggles to reclaim what deceit has taken away and still takes away. At the end of the book she describes being arrested for protesting at a nuclear test site. She and her fellow protesters are bused into the desert and left stranded. "What they didn't realize," Williams writes, "is that we were home." Her narrative wreckage is rebuilt; her map redrawn.

Four

The Restitution
Narrative

ILLNESS IN THE
IMAGINARY

The restitution narrative is the first of three types of narrative that I will propose. A narrative type is the most general story-line that can be recognized underlying the plot and tensions of particular stories. People tell their own unique stories, but they compose these stories by adapting and combining narrative types that cultures make available.

By a narrative type, I mean what a teller of folktales means when referring, for example, to a naming story. In the naming story, the protagonist has to guess the *true* name of the antagonist. The guessing counts because the antagonist threatens the protagonist; the antagonist's power can only be undone by speaking his true name. The protagonist may do the guessing himself if he is a trickster. Other protagonists need a helper, such as the mouse in the best-known naming story, the Grimm Brothers' "Rumpelstiltskin." Learning the value of the helper, whom the protagonist may initially reject, is a frequent sub-plot. Around the basic plot of the naming story all sorts of variations occur, just as naming can occur as a subplot in another story, but the narrative type remains identifiably within these variations.

My description of the naming story is not a random example of a narrative type. Although few would say it in these words, the teller of an illness story seeks to learn the true name of the disease, and perhaps her own true name as well. Nietzsche understood this, choosing to name his pain "dog."[1]

Why propose "types" of illness narratives and suggest that individual stories somehow "fit" one type or another? The risk is creating yet another "general unifying view" that subsumes the particularity of individual experience. The advantage is to encourage closer attention to the stories ill persons tell; ultimately, to aid listening to the ill. Listening is difficult because illness stories mix and weave different narrative threads. The rationale for proposing some general types of narratives is to sort out those threads.

My suggestion of three underlying narratives of illness does not deprecate the originality of the story any individual ill person tells, because no actual telling conforms exclusively to any of the three narratives. Actual tellings combine all three, each perpetually interrupting the other two. I limit myself to three basic narratives because if these types are to be used as *listening devices,* more than three seems less than helpful. Certainly, other types of narratives can and should be proposed.[2]

I consider each narrative type in four sections, beginning with its plot. Second, I describe the elective affinity that the narrative type has to the action problems of embodiment (control, body-relatedness, other-relatedness, and desire). Third is how the narrative works as a self-story. Finally I discuss the power of each narrative type and its limitations.

In any illness, *all* three narrative types are told, alternatively and repeatedly. At one moment in an illness, one type may guide the story; as the illness progresses, the story becomes told through other narratives. The particularity of any experiential moment can thus be described by the narrative type that predominates at that moment. The three narratives are like patterns in a kaleidoscope: for a moment the different colors are given one specific form, then the tube shifts and another form emerges. The retelling of illness stories, particularly the writing of oral stories, isolates the story of the moment from the narrative flux that marks lived storytelling. At the bedside, the kaleidoscope turns much more quickly than in print.

Each narrative reflects strong cultural and personal preferences. The strength of these preferences presents a further barrier to listening to the ill: both institutions and individual listeners steer ill people toward certain narratives, and other narratives are simply not heard. But barriers provide possibilities for insight. Reflection on one's own narrative preferences and discomforts is a moral problem, since in both listening to others and telling our own stories, we become who we are.

THE RESTITUTION PLOT

The restitution narrative dominates the stories of most people I talk to, particularly those who are recently ill and least often the chronically ill. Anyone who is sick wants to be healthy again. Moreover, contemporary culture treats health as the normal condition that people ought to have restored. Thus the ill person's own desire for restitution is compounded by the expectation that other people want to hear restitution stories.

The plot of the restitution has the basic storyline: "Yesterday I was healthy, today I'm sick, but tomorrow I'll be healthy again." This storyline is filled out with talk of tests and their interpretation, treatments and their possible outcomes, the competence of physicians, and alternative treatments. These events are real, but also they are metaphors in Schafer's sense of enacting the storyline of restoring health (see chapter 3). Metaphoric phrases like "as good as new" are the core of the restitution narrative. Such phrases are reflexive reminders of what the story is about: health.

Restitution stories can be told prospectively, retrospectively, and institutionally. I heard a prospective restitution story when

I met a man who, I had been told, was about to undergo surgery for cancer. I told him I was sorry to hear he was ill. He looked at me as if he was not sure what I was talking about and then, changing his expression to sudden recognition of what I referred to, immediately assured me it was "nothing." When we later spoke at length about his surgery, he told a story of how he would be able to assimilate various outcomes into his life without undo change. His prospective restitution story gave him the courage to face surgery. Later, following what turned out to be a long surgery and serious diagnosis, he might have needed a different story at a time when he lacked the energy to put one together.

I heard a retrospective restitution story one evening at a cancer support group. The group begins with a ritual that many groups use some variation of. Each person says his or her name, what kind of cancer he had, and when. Sometimes a bit of personal news is added. Most people close by saying, in a rising voice, "I'm fine!" Most regular group members are in remission from cancer, but this evening a woman attended who was currently in treatment. While she was describing the cancer she had, she broke into tears. The group response was for the person sitting next to her, the next speaker, to interrupt with her own introduction. She did this very briefly, moving to a particular emphasis on "I'm fine!" No one commented on the interruption or returned to acknowledge the distress of the person in treatment. Thus the group expressed its preference for restitution stories and its discomfort at hearing illness told in other narratives.

The restitution narrative not only reflects a "natural" desire to get well and stay well. People learn this narrative from institutional stories that model how illness is to be told. A major northeastern American hospital distributed an oversize tabloid newspaper supplement describing its cancer center. The brochure is sixteen pages long, printed on better than newsprint paper, and features obviously professional photography. Most of the content comprises the stories of three cancer patients. All three are told as restitution stories: "Within two weeks, Joan was back to work full-time," "Harry now has a new immune system that gives him every reason to believe it's a whole new ball game," and "Today, Mary has resumed her active, productive life—even adding a new pastime."

The brochure certainly fulfills a public education function, providing sidebar glossaries that clearly explain types of cancer and different treatments. But no patient is shown *in* treatment or affected by treatment. Photographs show patients pursuing their various "pastimes" of gardening, sports, and other hobbies. One radiotherapy machine is shown but not in use; the professional staff are posed sitting on it, as if having a conference. The patients' stories tell what their treatments were, but the emphasis is on life after treatment: returning to "I'm fine!"

Prospective patients reading this brochure are being educated not just about different cancers and their treatments. The brochure provides models of the stories patients ought to tell about their own illnesses. Institutional medicine is asserting its preferred narrative. This assertion goes beyond hospitals to the strategies that more powerful interest groups use to shape the culture of illness.

The most pervasive or, depending on one's values, the most insidious model of the restitution story is the television commercial for non-prescription drugs, frequently cold remedies. The plot unfolds in three movements. First, the ill person is shown in physical misery and, often though not always, in social default. Some activity with spouse or children is going to have to be canceled or work missed. The second movement introduces the remedy. As in the naming story, a helper may be involved in bringing the remedy, and also as in the naming story, a subplot may involve the sufferer's initial rejection of the remedy and thus of the helper. Eventually the remedy is taken, and the third movement shows physical comfort restored and social duties resumed. The success of the remedy validates the helper, and a hint of renewed romance may close the story.

To live in contemporary culture is to see such commercials without even noticing them; magazines can condense the plot to a single image, knowing that the reader/viewer will fill in the rest from memory. These advertisements set in place the narratives of the stories that real people tell about real illnesses. Commercials, like the hospital brochure described above, not only condition expectations for how sickness progresses; they also provide a model for how stories about sickness are told.

Here as elsewhere popular culture is most powerful when it reinforces habits of thought acquired elsewhere. The restitution plot is ancient: Job, after all his suffering, has his wealth and family restored, and whether or not that restoration was a later interpolation into the text, its place in the canonical version of the story shows the power of the restitution storyline. Television literally commercializes the Job story: the good person is suddenly struck down, but suffering is bourgeois (for example, a missed party or sports event), the remedy can be purchased, and the only learning involved is where to find relief next time.

Behind the hospital brochure and the commercial lies the modernist expectation that for every suffering there is a remedy. The consequences of this master narrative are complex. When the restitution ending is tacked onto Job, the nature of suffering changes from mystery to puzzle, to use a distinction from William May, who borrows from Gabriel Marcel.[3] A *mystery* can only be faced up to; a *puzzle* admits solution. The restitution ending of Job leaves the reader with the impression that somehow Job got it right, first in dialogue with his three friends and then in the whirlwind. The restitution is his prize for solving the puzzle, even if exactly how he solves it is not quite clear. Without the restitution, his suffering would remain a mystery, and a troubling one. The mystery cannot be solved, and while a person can seek to measure up to what a mystery presents, one cannot "get it right" because there is no "right" way to get it. This absence of solution makes mysteries a scandal to modernity.

Modernity seeks to turn mysteries into puzzles, which is both its heroism and its limit. Sociology, as one aspect of the modernist imagination, describes illness in its own restitution story, which is Talcott Parsons's theory of the "sick role," first presented in the early 1950s but elaborated throughout Parsons's career until his death in the late 1970s.[4] By a role, Parsons meant action that involves complementary expectations for behavior. Thus the "sick role" describes behavior the sick person expects from others and what they expect from him. These expectations are *institutionalized* in such matters as sick leave from work and medical care; they are validated by social *norms;* they are *functional* for society as a whole; and they are *internalized,* meaning that individuals regard their expectations around sickness as normal and natural.

Parsons makes three assumptions about the social meaning of illness. First, illness is not to be regarded as the sick person's fault. In an age that understands contagion and infection, becoming ill is not an indicator of moral failure but only the result some excessive stress, which Parsons perceived as both social and physiological. Second, the sick person is exempt from normal responsibilities, both at work and at home. Sick people can expect this exemption, and others have a reciprocal obligation to offer it. Third, because exemption from normal responsibilities requires social control lest its privilege be abused, the sick person is obligated to place himself under the authority of a recognized professional. Compliance to "doctor's orders" is fundamental to the social control aspect of the sick role; exemption is balanced by obligation.

Few social science students of medicine accept the sick role as a definitive description, but its narrative remains sufficiently compelling so that it can never be dismissed. I am not concerned here with the theory's empirical adequacy—for example, *are* most people excused from normal obligations when ill?—but rather with its force as a master narrative of restitution stories.

The sick role is a modernist narrative of social control. People become sick, in Parsons's view, when their normal obligations become overpowering or conflict with each other. Sickness is functional for society as an escape valve for excess social pressures. The problem of sickness from this functionalist perspective is how to give people sufficient time to recover without producing dropouts. Exemption must be granted, but it must also be regulated. The physician is explicitly a social control agent. For Parsons, one of the most important aspects of the physician's performance is refusing to "collude" with the patient; medical sympathy is to be limited by the overriding message that the sick person's task is to get well and return to normal obligations of work and family. The physician is there not to pander but to prod, gently but firmly.

Perhaps the central implicit assumption of the sick role, and what I believe provides its narrative force, is that people *do get well*, and many other people who do not get well want to continue to believe they will get well. To those whom I call members of the remission society, the sick role as Parsons describes it has little relevance. These people accept some level of illness as the permanent background and intermittent foreground of their lives. For Parsons, particularly the middle-aged Parsons who formulated the theory, any journey into the kingdom of illness is a limited one, from which return is both expected and possible.[5] The idea that the changing physical capabilities caused by sickness require ongoing renegotiation of social obligations and personal identity is not part of Parsons's theory.

Precisely because getting well is the only outcome Parsons

considers as acceptable, his theory of the sick role both reflects the assumptions of modernist medicine and inscribes the validity of these assumptions in a broader narrative of what society requires to function successfully. Whether or not the sick role describes the *experience* of being ill, and most agree it does not, it remains a powerful narrative of what medicine *expects from* the ill person and what other social institutions expect from medicine. At the core of those expectations is the assumption of restitution: returning the sick person to the status quo ante.

Behind the restitution narratives of popular culture and sociology is medicine. So much has been written about medicine's single-minded telos of cure that I will finesse quotation from some definitive clinical source and tell a mundane story. A physician friend told me, with distress, about his patient who is dying of cancer. The physician's distress is not from her dying; everyone dies, and many die too young. He hates watching his patient fall into a world of hospital specialists who refuse to accept that she is dying and continue to perform invasive tests that cannot lead to any viable treatment. Of course, it is his judgment that the treatment is futile, and the specialists might see the case differently.[6] But here was the same story, told so many times, being told again. Obsessed with cure, medicine cannot place the woman's story in any other narrative. Massive resources are expended, and, more important from the perspective of my physician friend, his patient is not being helped to find her way toward her own version of a good death. Medicine's hope of restitution crowds out any other stories.[7]

The restitution story, whether told by television commercials, sociology, or medicine, is the culturally preferred narrative. Nothing less is at stake in the viability of this narrative than the modernist project that Zygmunt Bauman calls "deconstructing mortality."[8] Modernity, Bauman argues, exorcises the fear of mortality by breaking down threats, among which illness is paradigmatic, into smaller and smaller units. To use May's distinction, the big mystery becomes a series of little puzzles. Medicine, with its division into specialties and sub-specialties, is designed to effect this deconstruction.[9]

When my mother-in-law, Laura Foote, was dying from cancer, we all knew she was dying. At least one reason why our family never talked about her dying was that until two days before she died we remained fixed on the incremental remedies that medicine continued to offer. However clear her deterioration, there was always another treatment option. As long as small puzzles could be solved, fixing this or medicating that, the big issue of mortality was evaded. Each specialist carried out his task with some success, and the patient died.

In its place, this deconstruction into small tasks can be therapeutic. When I was entering the hospital for my own recent biopsy, I found it mildly relieving to be subsumed in movements from one preoperative test to another; completing each form was a small victory, and I appreciated the distraction from my larger fear. But eventually the reality and responsibility of mortality, and its mystery, have to be faced. Doing so requires a story outside the restitution narrative.

THE RESTORABLE BODY

Although belief that the sufferings of illness will be relieved is always the preferred narrative for any body, some bodies show a greater affinity for restitution narratives than others. These bodies can be described using the dimensions of control, body-relatedness, other-relatedness, and desire. Because bodies do not stay put on these dimensions, affinity for the restitution narrative is a *stage in the embodiment process* of illness that every body passes through. When some variation of restitution is in the foreground of the person's story, it will be interrupted by other narratives, just as restitution interrupts these other narratives when they occupy the foreground.

On the control dimension, the teller of the restitution story wants the body's former *predictability* back again. This predictability is not simply the mechanical functioning that comes with a symptom-free life. What needs to be staved off is the deeper contingency represented by illness itself: the contingency of mortality. Any sickness is an intimation of mortality, and telling sickness as a restitution story forestalls that intimation.

But contingency is not so easily dispelled. The restitution is brought about by an agency outside the body: medicine operating through either surgery or drugs. The body's own contingency is remedied, but only by dependence on an agency that is other to the body. For the teller of restitution stories to consider the paradox—that this dependence institutes its own contingency—would spoil the restitution: in the television commercial the availability of the drug is unquestionable.

The body of the restitution story is fundamentally *monadic* in its relation to other bodies. The disease model of medicine reinforces this conception of each patient "having" a disease, and this disease model articulates well with modernist emphases on the individual as an autonomous entity. The same conception of the individual that makes it sensible to speak of "having" a disease can speak of "having" rights, "getting" an education, or, as will be discussed in the last chapters, "having" empathy. Diseases, rights, education, and empathy are seen as properties of specific persons, not as expressions of persons' relationships to others. Talk about "having" the disease turns the monadic body in upon itself.

The body that turns in upon itself is split from the self that looks forward to this body's restitution. The temporarily broken-down body becomes "it" to be cured. Thus the self is *dissociated* from the body. Both the TV commercial narrative and the sick-role narrative suggest the presence of a person inside the body who is affected by that body yet remains detached from it. The body is a kind of car driven around by the person inside; "it" breaks down and has to be repaired. The restitution story seems to say, "I'm fine but my body is sick, and it will be fixed soon." This story is a practice that supports and is supported by the modernist deconstruction of mortality: mortality is made a condition of the body, the body is broken down into discrete parts, any part can be fixed, and thus mortality is forestalled. Sickness as an intimation that my whole being is mortal is ruled out of consideration.

Finally, the body in restitution stories may be "it," but it wants to be cured; desire remains *productive*. What will cure the body is a commodity, whether that takes the form of a drug or a service, and however it is paid for. The TV commercial is a powerful master narrative not only as it instills the notion that for every ailment there is a remedy, but also because it shows the remedy as a packaged item to be purchased. Restitution is not only possible, it is *commodified*.

Commodification is a crucial aspect of the deconstruction of mortality: as long as I can buy this to fix that, I sustain an illusion of permanence. So long as there is more to buy, whatever needs fixing will be fixed, and I will continue to be. Lest this last mini-plot line seem exaggerated in its simplification, look in any newspaper for what Nicholas Regush, a medical investigative journalist, calls the "gee whiz" stories that pharmaceutical companies regularly send him for publication.[10] Whatever is wrong with the body, these stories describe the imminent development of a high-tech remedy that will cure it.

My sympathy for Regush's cynicism derives from having to sit through medical lectures that could only be called wildly enthusiastic as they proclaimed impending cures for cancer. If I have cancer again, I might seek these physicians and technologies, but another effect of the technologies—besides curing some people—is to imply that mortality itself is an avoidable contingency. Amid talk of the advances in genetic screening and manipulation, of drugs that can be delivered to the specific tumor site, and of new diagnostic imaging machines that detect pathology even earlier, amid all this restitution talk, the single certain fact of death has little place. The "gee whiz" news releases and medical self-congratulations are not wrong, but they betray a conspicuous lack of narrative balance: other stories are happening as well, and the restitution story crowds them out.

The body that predisposes choice of the restitution narrative, and the body that this narrative chooses, thus falls somewhere between the *disciplined body* and the *mirroring body*. The restitution story usually demands adherence to some regimen, and this medical (or alternative) compliance demands a disciplined body. But this body is also mirroring because of its emphasis on consumption. The restitution story is about remaking the body in an image derived either from its own history before illness or from elsewhere.

The mirroring body lives principally in what Lacan calls the realm of the Imaginary, where the self comprises images from elsewhere, layered upon each other to become that self. The reliance on images is obvious in the TV commercial: the "bad body" of sickness is juxtaposed with the "good body" of health, achieved after the remedy. The images presented for identification are clear. Identification is equally a central function of the physician in Parsons's sick role. The physician not only cures by his medicine, he also models health in his personal presence. The core of this "health" for Parsons is not the physician's own embodiment but his role performance. The physician is fulfilling the normal work obligations that the sick person has given up as he assumes the sick role. The image offered for the patient's identification is that of functioning worker.

The language of this last paragraph is filled with terms often used pejoratively: consumption as a mode of activity, identification with images, the primacy of work obligations. Against these pejorative connotations, I reiterate that the Imaginary as a mode of being is essential; self-identification in images only becomes neurotic when the individual lives *exclusively* in the Imaginary. Mirroring and disciplined bodies are perfectly appropriate modes of being; the problem, as with any mode of being, is becoming fixated in one of these bodies. The restitution story may be the first story I tell myself whenever I am ill, but I try to remind myself that other stories also have to be told.

RESTITUTION AS SELF-STORY

In the restitution story, the implicit genesis of illness is an unlucky breakdown in a body that is conceived on mechanistic lines. To be fixable, the body has to be a kind of machine. A Nobel prize-winning physician was interviewed in my morning paper. He suggested that for the reporter to understand his work, he should think of the body as a television set, and an elaborate analogy followed.[11] Restitution requires fixing, and fixing requires such a mechanistic view. The mechanistic view normalizes the illness: televisions break and require fixing, and so do bodies. The question of origin is subsumed in the puzzle of how to get the set working again.

This disinterest in genesis is typical of modernist thinking. Ernst Bloch wrote that modernists "do not seek legitimation in the original founding act, but in a future still to arrive."[12] The TV commercial does not consider how the person got sick in the first place; founding acts are effaced. Parsons does consider the forms of strain precipitating the sick role, but he does not discuss any need to change the conditions that gave rise to those strains. That the person in the sick role will return to the same conditions is not a consideration. As long as there is an infinite future of getting fixed, changing originating conditions seems irrelevant.

The absence of concern with genesis in restitution stories is clearest when other stories provide a contrast. The same morning newspaper that quoted the Nobel-winning cancer specialist also carried a feature on women suffering various ailments that they suspect result from leakage from silicon breast implants.[13] For these women, the "founding act" of having the initial implant is crucial: what they were told about the implants, what their surgeons knew, what the manufacturer knew, and why they had the surgery ("My self-esteem was low") are all reviewed in detail. But these, sadly, are not restitution stories; the women anticipate being sick for the rest of their lives and even passing that sickness on to their children.[14] When restitution is judged impossible, the founding act becomes crucial; when restitution is possible, the "future still to arrive" is preferred.

This preference for the future also affects how the interruption of illness is interpreted. Both the TV commercial and the sick role focus on sickness as interruption, but this interruption is finite and remediable. Restitution means that if there are any future interruptions, the sick person now knows the remedy that can fix them. The restitution narrative is a response to an interruption, but the narrative itself is above interruption. By contrast, the silicon breast implant story begins with a woman worrying whether her child's skin rash might be another result of silicon she believes he absorbed during breast feeding. Her worry is presented as an interjection that interrupts the questions the interviewer has been asking, just as the rash interrupts the woman's train of thought, just as the silicon-induced illnesses present a future of interminable interruptions. Her story is not a response to an interruption, but a narrative that is perpetually being interrupted.

The purpose that restitution narratives aim toward is two-fold. For the individual teller, the ending is a return to just before the beginning: "good as new" or status quo ante. For the culture that prefers restitution stories, this narrative affirms that breakdowns can be fixed. The remedy, now secure in the family medicine cabinet, becomes a kind of talisman against future sickness. One explanation for why Parsons does not consider the implication of returning the formerly sick person to the same conditions where he first became sick is that if sickness does return, the remedy can always be taken out of the cabinet, and the person can always go back to the doctor. In the extended logic of restitution, future sickness *already will have been cured.*

Just as the restitution narrative projects a future that will not be disrupted by illness, it also protects memory from disruption. In the restitution narrative, memory is not disrupted because the present illness is an aberration, a blip in the otherwise normal passage of time. The "normal" trajectory remains intact. After I had cancer I saw a colleague who had been on leave during my illness. He was most solicitous about what had happened to me, and finally mentioned that he himself had had cancer once, but it hadn't amounted to much. As we talked it developed he actually had the same cancer I had, a testicular tumor, but while his was found early and operated on immediately, I suffered from misdiagnosis and extensive secondary tumors.

Our diagnostic differences were equally narrative differences. His story had turned into a restitution narrative before he had time to tell it any other way. His memory of cancer was something remembered outside of memory, insofar as memory involves placing experiences into patterns, albeit changing patterns. He remembered cancer, but cancer was scarcely part of any pattern of recollection. For the teller of the restitution story, sickness is not memorable, though restitution may be, especially if it is exceptional. Restitution makes a good story after the fact only if it was unexpected.

My colleague's cancer experience was over in a couple of weeks. For that incident to have crystallized any significant issues of responsibility would have been unusual, though this also happens. A woman who has made a vocation of her volunteer work for our local cancer society explains her commitment, in emotional terms, by describing a cancer scare she had. She was investigated for a condition that turned out not to be cancer and, so far as I know, has not caused her health problems since. But she was intimate with a family whose lives were determined over many years by the cancer and eventual death of the mother. That intimacy gave her cancer scare a narrative context, and thus a force, that the actual cancer of my colleague never acquired. Her experience left her with a heavy sense of responsibility; she joined Schweitzer's community of those who bear the mark of pain. Even though the medical facts of her case fit a restitution model, her narrative is not one of restitution.

The issue of responsibility suggests one of the crucial differences between types of narrative: the difference concerning what sort of agency the narrative affords the ill person. In the restitution narrative, the responsibility is limited to taking one's medicine and getting well, wellness being defined in contrast to illness. Other narratives understand the experience of illness in a way that makes returning to the same life that was lived before illness impossible as a moral choice. Schweitzer expressed this when he wrote that whoever "has learned what pain and anxiety really are must help to ensure that those out there who are in physical need obtain the same help that once came to him."[15]

Schweitzer is positing a restoration to health, but not within a restitution narrative. Life for the person Schweitzer describes has changed fundamentally, even though illness is cured. Responsibility is based on an ongoing sense of solidarity with the ill, this solidarity transcending the present health or illness of one's own body.

Is the restitution narrative capable of generating self-stories? No, in the sense that restitution stories bear witness not to the struggles of the self but to the expertise of others: their competence and their caring that effect the cure. In this witness restitution stories reveal themselves to be told *by* a self but not *about* that self. The self of the mirroring body is realized in identifications with images of others; the witness of the restitution story can only be to the validity of those images.

But this "no" must be qualified by recognizing that not every illness story has to be a self-story; even among the seriously ill, many people do not have their sense of coherence disrupted. Little is perceived as having been taken away, so what is there to reclaim? Consciousness has remained sovereign over its experience. The restitution narrative has its proper sphere: images of health can model behavior that many people can adopt and adapt. The problem arises when the ill person does not find restitution, or when someone who can only tell restitution stories encounters another whose health will not be restored.

THE POWER AND LIMITATIONS OF RESTITUTION

Restitution stories are compelling because they often are true: many people do exit the kingdom of illness, sooner than later, good as new. The cultural power of these stories is that their telling reflects one of the best impulses in modernity: the heroism of applied science as self-overcoming. Robert Zussman, summarizing his study of medical work in intensive care units, coins the phrase "the banality of heroism." "If [medical house-staff] are heroic," Zussman writes, "they are heroic in the routine course of doing their jobs, preparing for the future, and getting through the day."[16]

Ill people who tell restitution stories practice their own banality of heroism. They live out illness as a matter of doing their jobs as patients, preparing for the future after illness, and getting through their own days. The restitution story, precisely because it treats sickness as banal, displays a heroism in the face of bodily breakdown. But this heroism of the ill person is invariably tied to the more active heroism of the healer.

The respective heroisms of physicians and patients are complementary but asymmetrical. Each heroism is required by the other, but physicians practice an active heroism, while patients accept a passive heroism. This asymmetry is not a problem—it may be the only sensible arrangement—but the ill person who adopts this narrative as his own self-story thereby accepts a place in a moral order that subordinates him as an individual.

This subordination is implied in Zussman's observation that physicians' sense of responsibility is not to patients so much as it is to other physicians. He goes on to refer to house-staff valuing medicine as "an encapsulated intellectual challenge." Zussman is well aware that not all patients will appreciate the physicians' values of collegial responsibility or encapsulation, but these values are nevertheless "of primary importance to the profession of medicine."[17]

Zussman's insightful depiction of medical heroism can be placed in a larger perspective by Bauman's distinction between the modernist "hero" and the postmodern "moral person."[18] The hero believes in a cause that is "nobler, loftier, more worthy than their own self-preservation." What Zussman describes as "the profession of medicine" assumes the stature of such a cause; he makes it clear that the comfort and often the safety of both patients and physicians are worth risking. "The profession of medicine" could easily join Bauman's list of mod-

ernist causes that are "the continuation or promotion or triumph of an idea: that of a nation, of a race, of a class, or a 'way of
life', of God, sometimes of 'man as such'" (209).

Across the postmodern divide and in contrast to the hero,
Bauman's "moral person" takes as his cause "the life or well-
being or dignity of another human being" (209). The moral
person would risk neither himself nor anyone in his care for
such an idea as "the profession of medicine." If an idea does
not respect the value and dignity of any immediate person, if it
demands the person be sacrificed, then it is not an idea worth
respecting. But that is a postmodern attitude.[19]

Restitution stories inscribe a modernist narrative both in illness experience and in medical treatment. The first limitation
of restitution stories is the obvious but often neglected limitation of the modernist deconstruction of mortality: when it
doesn't work any longer, there is no other story to fall back on.
Restitution stories no longer work when the person is dying or
when impairment will remain chronic. When restitution does
not happen, other stories have to be prepared or the narrative
wreckage will be real.

Sherwin Nuland, writing as a senior physician who has attended many deaths, evokes the "final sharing" that can snatch
"an enduring comfort and even some dignity from the an-
guished fact of death."[20] Nuland castigates his medical colleagues whose adherence to an ideal of cure robs dying
persons and their families of this sharing. What he calls "the
seduction of The Riddle" (249) is what I call being captured by
the exclusivity of the restitution narrative. This narrative leaves
no place for stories that will disencumber the dying person of
what Nuland describes as "the baggage we shall all take to the
grave": "unresolved, breached relationships not healed, potential unfulfilled, promises not kept, and years that will never be
lived" (261). Even the very old, Nuland observes, do not always
escape having this unfinished business.

Nuland asserts a stronger version of responsibility than any other medical commentator. "The dying themselves," he writes, "bear a responsibility not to be entrapped by a misguided attempt to spare those whose lives are intertwined with theirs" (243). The restitution narrative can be just such a trap.

Another limitation, perhaps opposite to the above, is that restitution is increasingly a commodity that some can purchase and others cannot. Imagine the person watching the TV commercial who has the same ailment but no money to buy the remedy. High-tech medicine offers more and more restitutions that fewer and fewer people will be able to afford.[21] Thus the restitution story as a *generalized* narrative of illness can be predicted to become increasingly restricted in its availability.

But even if medical progress will be limited in whom it benefits, this progress is real and remains the ultimate power of the restitution narrative. The ultimate limitation of restitution is mortality: the confrontation with mortality cannot be part of the story. Sometimes what cannot be told is dramatic, as when my physician friend cannot wrest his patient from specialists and discuss her imminent death with her. Other times nothing prohibits talking about death, but something just as strong inhibits this talk.

Zygmunt Bauman, responding to arguments presented by Norbert Elias, describes why the restitution narrative is inadequate to make mortality available to experience. "Perhaps it is not just the delicacy of manner that deprives us of speech [when we encounter the dying]," Bauman writes, "but also the simple fact that, indeed, we have nothing to say to a person who has no further use for the *language of survival;* a person who is about to leave the world of busy pretense that that language conjures up and sustains."[22]

Professional medicine, on the sociological accounts of Parsons, Zussman, and other students of its practices, and on the practitioner accounts of physicians like Nuland, institutionalizes having nothing to say beyond the language of survival. Its studied self-restriction to that language is the core of its banality of heroism. This core shows widening cracks in postmodern times. Many physicians seem less interested in being heros, in Bauman's modernist sense, and more interested in being moral persons. Nuland's self-reflections, and their enormous popular reception, are one indication of this shift; David Hilfiker, in his life as well as his writing, is another.[23]

My interest, however, is less in forecasting medical change and more in what happens to ill people. What happens when those who have always spoken their own experience in the language of survival find that language has nothing left to say about themselves, once the viability of restitution has run out? What body-self is left, when the end of survival is imminent? The tragedy is not death, but having the self-story end before the life is over. It is a tragedy if having nothing else to say means that these people have no further use for themselves; if in Audre Lorde's phrase they have lost any language in which they can remain available to themselves. Living can certainly be more than the "life of busy pretense," and stories are available that conjure up these other possibilities. But before describing stories that affirm life beyond restitution, the stories that deny any possibility of restitution must be heard.

Five

The Chaos Narrative

Mute Illness

Chaos as Non-Plot

Chaos is the opposite of restitution: its plot imagines life never getting better. Stories are chaotic in their absence of narrative order. Events are told as the storyteller experiences life: without sequence or discernable causality. The lack of any coherent sequence is an initial reason why chaos stories are hard to hear; the teller is not understood as telling a "proper" story. But more significantly, the teller of the chaos story is not heard to be living a "proper" life, since in life as in story, one event is expected to lead to another. Chaos negates that expectation.

Chaos stories are as anxiety provoking as restitution stories are preferred. Telling chaos stories represents the triumph of all that modernity seeks to surpass. In these stories the modernist bulwark of remedy, progress, and professionalism cracks to reveal vulnerability, futility, and impotence. If the restitution narrative promises possibilities of outdistancing or outwitting suffering, the chaos narrative tells how easily any of us could be sucked under. Restitution stories reassure the listener that however bad things look, a happy ending is possible—Job with his new family and cattle, basking in God's graciousness. Chaos stories are Job taking his wife's advice, cursing God and dying.

Chaos stories are also hard to hear because they are too

threatening. The anxiety these stories provoke inhibits hearing. Like many people, I saw the chaotic side of illness experience for years before I could acknowledge it. To hear what was being told, I needed the distance of other stories telling events that were not only outside my own experience, but outside the topic of illness. I first began to hear the chaos narrative in Holocaust stories and commentary on them.[1] What cannot be evaded in stories told by Holocaust witnesses is the hole in the narrative that cannot be filled in, or to use Lacan's metaphor, cannot be sutured. The story traces the edges of a wound that can only be told around. Words suggest its rawness, but that wound is so much of the body, its insults, agonies, and losses, that words necessarily fail.

The teller of chaos stories is, preeminently, the wounded storyteller, but those who are truly *living* the chaos cannot tell in words. To turn the chaos into a verbal story is to have some reflective grasp of it. The chaos that can be told in story is already taking place at a distance and is being reflected on retrospectively. For a person to gain such a reflective grasp of her own life, distance is a prerequisite. In telling the events of one's life, events are mediated by the telling. But in the lived chaos there is no mediation, only immediacy. The body is imprisoned in the frustrated needs of the moment. The person living the chaos story has no distance from her life and no reflective grasp on it. Lived chaos makes reflection, and consequently storytelling, impossible.

If narrative implies a sequence of events connected to each other through time, chaos stories are not narratives. When I refer below to the chaos narrative, I mean an *anti-narrative* of time without sequence, telling without mediation, and speaking about oneself without being fully able to reflect on oneself. Although I will continue to write of chaos stories as being told, these stories cannot literally be told but can only be lived.

Yet if the chaotic story cannot be told, the voice of chaos can be identified and a story reconstructed. What this voice sounds like is captured in an interview fragment reported by Kathy Charmaz. The speaker, Nancy, is a woman with a chronic illness as well as multiple family problems. She describes living with her mother who has Alzheimer's; her mother, she says, "just won't leave me alone."

> And if I'm trying to get dinner ready and I'm already feeling bad, she's in front of the refrigerator. Then she goes to put her hand on the stove and I got the fire on. And then she's in front of the microwave and then she's in front of the silverware drawer. And— and if I send her out she gets mad at me. And then it's awful. That's when I have a really, a really bad time.[2]

Hearing the story in Nancy's talk is not easy. First, the story has no narrative sequence, only an incessant present with no memorable past and no future worth anticipating. Second, this anti-narrative contains nothing but life possibilities that anyone fears precisely because almost anyone could end up living in conditions like Nancy's.

Nancy's story displays the chaos narrative in at least two other respects as well. First is the overdetermination of her situation. Nancy is "already feeling bad" from her own illness as she has to contend with her mother. The overdetermination of her problems extends to her troubles with children, dogs, insurance bureaucracies, and, the listener comes to wonder, *who knows what else.* In the chaos narrative, troubles go all the way down to bottomless depths. What can be told only begins to suggest all that is wrong.

The second feature of chaos narrative in Nancy's story is the syntactic structure of "and then and then and then." This staccato pacing of words pecks away at the reader just as Nancy's life pecks away at her. In chaos stories, the untellable silence alternates with the insistent "and then" repetitions. The personal and cultural dislike for such stories—a dislike that takes the form of simply being unable to hear the story—becomes self-evident.

Gilda Radner's story of her treatment for ovarian cancer is not a chaos narrative, precisely because it is a narrative. But Radner allows readers some vision of the chaos. Radner is not Nancy; she does have space for reflection; she is writing. The chaos in her life occurs during chemotherapy when the sleeping pills Radner takes cause her to forget, completely, whatever has happened: "Even if I'd gotten sick from the chemo, I wouldn't remember."[3] She hates the loss of these days, the literal hole they create in her life. One creative response is to videotape her chemotherapy (169–79). She may miss the world as it goes on around her, but at least she can see what happened to herself. The tape fills in part of the hole in her life; chaos is retrospectively remediated. The story of the videotaping is not the chaos; the story is told around the edges of that hole.

The deeper issue for Radner is the loss of control in her life; time lost during chemotherapy, real enough in itself, also represents this greater loss. "The issue of control plagued me," she writes; " despite the war I was waging, and my endurance, I couldn't control the outcome" (181). Control and chaos exist at opposite ends of a continuum. The restitution story presupposes the control that is necessary to effect restitution. The ill person does not have this control herself, but those taking care of her do, which for the restitution story is close enough. The chaos story presupposes *lack* of control, and the ill person's loss of control is complemented by medicine's inability to control the disease.

Chaos feeds on the sense that *no one* is in control. People living these stories regularly accuse medicine of seeking to maintain its pretense of control—its restitution narrative—at the expense of denying the suffering of what it cannot treat.

Endometriosis, although recognized as a disease, is often experienced when it cannot be diagnosed. Sally Golby describes her struggle to gain medical recognition of her endometriosis: "The fact the doctors were ignorant about the disease is an excuse, but the fact they battered me emotionally is not."[4] The present issue is not the difficulty of diagnosing a disease like endometriosis, or the contested reality of conditions like chronic fatigue syndrome (which sufferers prefer to call myalgic encephalomyelitis, in part to display greater diagnostic credibility). The issue is the sense that Sally Golby has of being battered: that emotional battering is fundamental to chaos.

When somehow some part of the chaos is told, no one wants to hear. Lawrence Langer, studying the recordings of oral histories of the Holocaust, observed how interviewers undercut the stories that the surviving witnesses were telling. Very subtly the interviewers direct witnesses toward another narrative that exhibits "the resiliency of the human spirit."[5] The human spirit certainly is resilient, but Langer forces his readers to recognize that *that is not what the witnesses are saying.* When Nancy tells about her troubles with her mother, we can hear the resilience of the human spirit, but Nancy herself is trying to get recognition of the utter chaos of her life.

The challenge of encountering the chaos narrative is how not to steer the storyteller away from her feelings, as Langer shows the interviewers of Holocaust witnesses doing. The challenge is to *hear.* Hearing is difficult not only because listeners have trouble facing what is being said as a possibility or a reality in their own lives. Hearing is also difficult because the chaos narrative is probably the most embodied form of story. If chaos stories are told on the edges of a wound, they are also told on the edges of speech. Ultimately, chaos is told in the silences that speech cannot penetrate or illuminate.

The chaos narrative is always beyond speech, and thus it is what is always *lacking* in speech. Chaos is what can never be told; it is the hole in the telling. Thus in the most hurried "and then" telling, chaos is the ultimate muteness that forces speech to go faster and faster, trying to catch the suffering in words.

CHAOS EMBODIED

The chaotic body can be described in terms of the dimensions of control, body- and other-relatedness, and desire, but the resulting permutation does not fit any of the four ideal types suggested in chapter 2, thus showing that while those types illustrate certain parameters of body-selves, they certainly do not circumscribe reality.

On the control dimension, the body telling chaos stories defines itself as being swept along, without control, by life's fundamental *contingency*. Efforts to reassert predictability have failed repeatedly, and each failure has had its costs. Contingency is not exactly accepted; rather, it is taken as inevitable. Denials of the chaos narrative often begin with the listener asserting how, in such circumstances, he would find some way out. Primo Levi describes telling his concentration camp experiences to a group of school children, and one boy responding with a detailed plan of how he could have escaped.[6] My equivalent experiences take place in odd conversations—both strange and mercifully infrequent—when someone who has never had cancer tells me about psychological changes they have made in their lives that are going to protect them from this disease. All of us on the outside of some chaos want assurances that if we fell in, *we* could get out. But the chaos narrative is beyond such bargaining; there is no way out.

Relationships also have a history of failure, and so in terms of other-relatedness, the body is *monadic*. This monadic orientation contributes to the inability to find recognition or support for the body's pain and suffering. A feedback loop is initiated: chaos stories erect a wall around the teller that prevents her from being assisted or comforted, and the less assistance and comfort she experiences, the more she may feel compelled to breach that wall with monologues that repeat "and then."[7]

The incapacity to receive comfort both reflects and reinforces the body's *lack* of desire. Whatever desires it once had have been too frequently frustrated. In a world so permeated by contingencies that turn out badly, desire is not only pointless but dangerous, just as relationships with others have become dangerous.

Association with one's own body is also dangerous. The body is so degraded by an overdetermination of disease and social mistreatment that survival depends on the self's *dissociation* from the body, even while the body's suffering determines whatever life the person can lead. But matters are more complex than a "self" dissociating itself from a body. A person who has recently started to experience pain speaks of "it" hurting "me" and can dissociate from that "it." The chaos narrative is lived when "it" has hammered "me" out of self-recognition. Chaos stories are told at the end of the process that Elaine Scarry calls "unmaking the world."[8]

Nancy's world is unmade. As her chaos story describes her mother in the kitchen, Nancy herself becomes a null point around which her mother moves. The physical space of the kitchen surrounds Nancy, but what is eerie in her description is that Nancy does not move through this space; instead, she is there only as obstructed. Reduced to being an occasion for obstruction, Nancy's body has lost any agency. She is the disembodied subject of a story that she nominally tells but that contains nothing of her subjectivity. Thus Nancy's story is frenzied but flat; she can no longer express sadness at what her life has become.

The skill of the interviewer, Kathy Charmaz, is to elicit an evocation of Nancy's chaos. The reader hears what can rarely be heard: the unmaking of a person's world. What haunts the reader is hearing Nancy fade into a voice that speaks only its own interruptions: all the "and then" contingencies that fragment her story and her life.

gum

Contingent, monadic, lacking desire, and dissociated—such is the configuration of traits that typify the *chaotic body.* It is often victim to dominating bodies, which make it the object of their force. It is scandal to mirroring bodies, since it shows how easily the images they use to construct themselves can be stripped away. To the disciplined body, the chaotic body represents weakness and inability to resist. The dominating, mirroring, and disciplined bodies each suppress the possibility that they could become chaotic; the chaotic body is the other against which these bodies define themselves. But they claim no empathic relation to this body; it represents only what they fear for themselves.

For the communicative body, the chaotic body is the traveler whom the Good Samaritan found robbed and beaten by the roadside. The communicative body also defines itself through the chaotic body, but the chaotic body is not other to it. Rather, the communicative body sees itself in the chaotic body, and finds inescapable the gesture of offering itself to that body.[9] Note that for most mortals this gesture requires limits: even the Samaritan goes on about his business, paying the inn keeper to care for the injured man. This chapter, however, is more concerned with the tragedy of the chaotic body: of the one whose world is so unmade that he cannot accept the Samaritan's gift.

THE CHAOTIC SELF-STORY

In the chaos narrative, consciousness has given up the struggle for sovereignty over its own experience. When such a struggle can be told, then there is some distance from the chaos; some part of the teller has emerged. Thus just as the chaos narrative is an anti-narrative, so it is a non-self-story. Where life can be given narrative order, chaos is already at bay. In stories told out of the deepest chaos, no sense of sequence redeems suffering as orderly, and no self finds purpose in suffering.

Nancy is not only too frequently interrupted to be able to write her story down; her story is too interrupted to be susceptible to being written. Gilda Radner, although her disease is terminal, can secure an uninterrupted space—physical and psychological—to write her story. The interruption posed by cancer and each of its recurrences is overridden by the story she tells: cancer can interrupt her life, but as she turns those interruptions into a coherent story, she neutralizes the chaos immanent in them. Radner's ability to keep writing her story, mustering all the resources that writing requires, separates her from Nancy's chaos.

The difference between Nancy and Gilda Radner represents the paradox that a true chaos story cannot be told. The voice that might express deepest chaos is subsumed in interruptions, interrupting itself as it seeks to tell. This self-interruption is the core of the "and then" style of speech, cutting off each clause with the next.

The interruptions undercut any pursuit of purpose, and if there were a sense of purpose, again the story would not be chaos. In his analysis of how interviewers elicit Holocaust stories, Langer notes that one device they use to keep the talk tolerable for themselves is to steer the witness toward what the interviewer takes as the end of the camp experience, liberation; liberation becomes the closest thing to a purpose that can redeem the horror. But witnesses, unlike their interviewers, do not think of liberation as any great dividing line that orders their experience. Most striking is one witness whom Langer quotes. In response to being asked how he felt about liberation

he says, "Then I knew my troubles were *really* about to begin."
Langer points out that this statement inverts expectations
grounded in "traditional historical narrative."[10]

The witness's statement recalls Oliver Sacks's story about his
last night in a London hospital where his badly injured leg has
been repaired. Sacks's troubles began when he injured himself
in a hiking accident.[11] Surgery on his leg is successful from a
medical perspective, but Sacks has no sensation in the leg. The
problem is not just failure of the nerves to feel and respond.
The deeper problem is that Sacks sees his own leg as not being
his. He describes the leg as feeling "meaningless and unreal
. . . an absolutely ludicrous artificial leg."[12] Nurses and orthopedic surgeons refuse to acknowledge any aspect of what Sacks
is experiencing, and their denial increases his "horrible fears
and phantasms" (127). Sacks's chaos is his extreme dissociation
from what he knows is part of his body but cannot experience
as belonging to himself.

Sacks regains sensation in his leg by listening to Mendelssohn; internalizing the rhythms of the music, he begins to
walk again. Eventually he is to be discharged from the hospital
to a kind of halfway house for rehabilitation. His moment of
deepest chaos would seem to be behind him. His story's narrative has become one of recovery, yet he was, as he puts it, "dead
scared of leaving." In his fear I hear an echo, however faint, of
"my troubles were *really* about to begin."

The hospital's time and space have come to circumscribe
Sacks's world. On his last night in this world he decides to
climb up onto the hospital roof, on crutches with his leg still in
a cast, to see the view of London at night. Fortunately a nurse
stops him before the inevitable accident occurs. Later he
learns how many patients engage in similar attempts to sabo-
tage their imminent releases (166). The manic humor of
Sacks's tale of this escapade rests on an edge of terror, though
terror of *what?*

Too quick explanations of "fear of reentry" trivialize what Sacks faced. He had known chaos and been face to face with his own dissolution. His fear is of reentering a world that cannot imagine, and does not want to imagine, that dissolution. This reentry is a worse trouble than language can readily formulate.

Many people with cancer report a kind of terror when the treatments they have hated finally end, usually explaining this as a fear of recurrence.[13] That explanation, with its emphasis on cure, turns their stories into restitution narratives. Yet Sacks seems to reject restitution in his desire to climb back into darkness: if not the darkness of his original injury, then at least the darkness of the roof with its probability of accident and continued hospitalization.

At various times during my own treatment for cancer I both hated the hospital and found it was the only place where I felt I had a place. Chemotherapy was both the proximate source of my chaos and a sort of solution to the problem it itself generated. That solution was *not* getting to the end of treatment. The solution was being kept apart from a world that could not, and would not, understand. When liberation from the hospital comes, as welcome as it is, one's real trouble begins: the trouble of remaking a sense of purpose as the world demands.

Parsons labeled ill people as seeking a "secondary gain" when they remain in the "sick role" longer than they apparently need to. Gains include benefits such as attention, care, and excuse from other responsibilities. Such an explanation, applied by healthy analysts to ill people, is a bit like the clock that has stopped but is still correct twice a day. Something is explained, but the whole notion of "explaining" requires imposing a purpose on behavior. Much illness behavior can only be understood when the would-be interpreter is able to enter imaginatively into a world *without* purpose. The interviewers described by Langer seek to impose liberation as, if not a goal, then at least a definite end to the stories they hear and the horrors these stories tell. The Holocaust witness who resists this narrative imposition inverts the narrative order by showing the interviewer the inapplicability of finding any ending in liberation.

When Sacks captures his moments of chaos in prose, he writes from well outside a chaos that the Holocaust witness can never leave behind. Sacks's story invokes moments of chaos, but it is hardly a chaos narrative. Sacks tells a series of interruptions—first his accident, then the post-surgical lack of feeling in his leg, then his misadventure on the roof, and so on—but these interruptions are assimilated into a stable pattern of memory. In Sacks's story, one thing leads to another. To the extent that such a narrative ordering can be discovered and told, beginning with a clear *genesis,* that story seems to keep the body out of chaos.[14] A sense of genesis sets in place subsequent narrative order: something early results in something else later on.

The Holocaust stories may have a clear historical genesis, the moment of being transported to the camp, but in the depths of all that happens later, this moment loses narrative force as an explanation. In a chaos story such as Nancy's, the genesis of her troubles is lost in the overdetermination of these troubles: which came first—illness, financial problems, family problems—is impossible to sort out. The lack of genesis in chaos stories has its corresponding lack in any sense of the future. Thus the chaos narrative shows the truth of Carr's observation (see chapter 3) that a coherent whole requires all three: future, present, and past, each depending on the others. In a story such as Nancy's, which lack precedes which—past or future—cannot be told.

Just as a story of chaos cannot be told from within the chaos, the responsibility implied by an experience of chaos cannot be exercised from within the chaos. The person who has lived chaos can only be responsible to that experience retrospectively, when distance allows reflection and some narrative ordering of temporality. The body-self that is immersed in a chaos lives only in immediacy. Whenever events seem to be sorted out, the chaos generates another crisis of survival.

Exercising responsibility requires a *voice,* and the chaotic body has no voice; I imagine Nancy cannot hear her voice as entirely her own. Muteness begins in the body; when Sacks cannot experience a part of his body as part of himself, he cannot speak, at least in the sense of articulating his feelings in a way that gains the recognition of others. His story suggests how speech requires the body that is spoken through: Sacks is unable to speak through his body when it seems only contingently attached to him. The achievement of his writing is to capture the claustrophobic terror of this muteness.

Sacks is awakened from this nightmare by Mendelssohn. Music allows a direct connection to his body that speech can no longer provide. As he learns to turn musical rhythms into movement, Sacks begins—the story does not end here—to rediscover the use of this body and thus reintegrate himself. Eventually he finds a voice to witness his experience— ultimately in his book—but this voice can only speak *about* the chaos, from *outside* that chaos. Being a mute witness, caught within the chaos itself, is a condition of horror.

HONORING THE CHAOS STORY

The need to honor chaos stories is both moral and clinical. Until the chaos narrative can be honored, the world in all its possibilities is being denied. To deny a chaos story is to deny the person telling this story, and people who are being denied cannot be cared for. People whose reality is denied can remain recipients of treatments and services, but they cannot be participants in empathic relations of care. The chaotic body is disabled with respect to entering relationships of care; as suggested above, it cannot tell enough of its own story to formulate its needs and ask for help; often it cannot even accept help when it is offered.

Those living chaotic stories certainly need help, but the immediate impulse of most would-be helpers is first to drag the teller out of this story, that dragging called some version of "therapy." Getting out of chaos is to be desired, but people can only be helped out when those who care are first willing to become witnesses to the story. Chaos is never transcended but must be accepted before new lives can be built and new stories told. Those who care for lives emerging from chaos have to accept that chaos always remains the story's background and will continually fade into the foreground.

The exemplary fortitude of Oliver Sacks, the man with the unreal leg, is to refuse to play the role of doctor to himself, even though he is a doctor. Against medical denial that anything is wrong, Sacks sticks with his perception, as fearful as that is. He stays in his body until it finds its own way out of the chaos, which for him begins through music.

The worst thing medical staff can do to someone in the chaos story is rush him to move on. Moving on is desirable; chaos is the pit of narrative wreckage. But attempting to push the person out of this wreckage only denies what is being experienced and compounds the chaos. The anxiety that the chaos story provokes in others leads to the standard clinical dismissal of chaos stories as documenting "depression." When chaos is thus redefined as a treatable condition, the restitution narrative is restored. Clinical staff can once again be comfortably in control: the chaos can be dismissed as the patient's personal malfunction. That reality is classified as either amenable or resistant to treatment; in either case it no longer represents an existential threat.[15]

What is needed, specifically in clinical work and more generally in any interpersonal relations, is an enhanced tolerance for chaos as a part of a life story. Robert Bly cites Norwegian scholars who write about medieval customs of young men dropping out, sometimes for two or three years, to lie in the ashes of the fire pits in the large, communal houses. "Apparently some also chewed cinders," Bly notes, explaining their name of Cinder-Biters.[16] Bodies living chaos stories are contemporary Cinder-Biters.

I worry that this chapter has already drawn too many analogies between forms of suffering that cannot be compared. Unlike the Cinder-Biters, Nancy is not going through a developmental phase as she attempts to cope with her chronic illness, her mother's Alzheimer's, and her other problems. But a society that had an accepted place for Cinder-Biters might show more empathy for Nancy's condition and be able to provide for more of her needs. Nancy would have a recognized place in such a society, while she has no place in ours. Because contemporaries, whether medical or lay, cannot allow themselves to imagine her chaos—to entertain it as anything close to their normality—they can only pile more sickness labels on her, driving her deeper into chaos.

Here as elsewhere, the clinical problem reflects a larger social issue. Clinicians cannot entertain chaos because chaos is an implicit critique of the modernist assumptions of clinical work. Reconsider that provocative, Zen koan-like line of the Holocaust witness describing liberation, "Then I knew my troubles were *really* about to begin." What is inverted here are not just the expectations of historical narrative, but the modernist understanding of history, both social and personal, as progress. When interviewers steer witnesses toward liberation, they reinstitute a modernist restitution narrative of progress. The great modernist exemplars of my own youth were the Japanese and German "economic miracles" of rebuilding and, as a kind of complementary phenomenon, the creation of Israel. After Auschwitz and Hiroshima, these phenomena restored faith in the modernist project.

Many intellectuals—Theodor Adorno, Maurice Blanchot, Edmond Jabes, Jean-François Lyotard—have asked how it is possible to write after Auschwitz. Perhaps the other question that ought to be asked is how it was possible to write before: what naivete informed modernity from its inception? The immediate relevance of this question is that the same naivete continues to suppress the chaos story. Clinical caregivers steer patients toward medical versions of liberation: treatment plans, rehabilitation, functional normality, lifestyle counseling, remission. These phrases and the many others like them reinstitute the restitution narrative. My objective is hardly to romanticize chaos; it is horrible. But modernity has a hard time accepting, even provisionally, that life sometimes *is* horrible. The attendant denial of chaos only makes its horror worse.

This horror is a mystery that can only be faced, never solved. Working out treatment plans and seeking to achieve remissions are fine, heroic work, in the perspective of what they are. The serious question is whether the heroic work of modernity, exemplified by Zussman's intensive care physicians, can proceed in concert with the kind of tragic consciousness that affords a normal place to Cinder-Biters: a consciousness that does not see these people as in need of fixing but honors them for what they are being.

Much of postmodernity—haunted by the question of how to write after Auschwitz—is a struggle to work out what aspects of modernity can be preserved while scrapping the modernist telos. In this telos the restitution narrative demands hegemony; it denies chaos and requires chaotic bodies to be "depressed" and thus fixable. There is no modernist clinical category for "living a life of overwhelming trouble and suffering," yet only this label can describe someone like Nancy being buffeted about her kitchen, or the Holocaust witness, or Gilda Radner as she goes through recurrence after recurrence of cancer, or Oliver Sacks as he looks at his leg and cannot see it as part of his body.

Sacks's chaos has its macrocosmic analogue when society looks at people in chaos and cannot see them as part of the social body. The difference is that Sacks takes it as his problem to reclaim his leg; society often attributes the problem to these "others" themselves. The most prevalent North American example of these others are the homeless. As ill persons, the homeless present an ambiguity: Hilfiker writes of the poorest sections of Washington, D.C. that "health is not so much a question of disease."[17] Hilfiker evokes the inversion of Parsons's sick role: lives of sickness outside medical purview. "The strictly medical factors are rarely the most crucial to healing," he observes (211). His diagnosis is what I call "living a life of overwhelming trouble and suffering." Society prefers medical diagnoses that admit treatment, not social diagnoses that require massive change in the premises of what that social body includes as parts of itself.[18]

The very poor and the very sick have only a marginal place in the case load of the professions, which prefer what can be fixed. Hilfiker describes how this preference is enforced in medical schools. After a lecture he gives, a "distinguished professor of pediatric surgery, garbed in a long white coat" rises to ask him whether his practice of poverty medicine is not a "waste" of his medical education. Hilfiker acknowledges having little opportunity in his conditions of practice to exercise his scientific skills. He also recognizes that the professor is using the question to "persuade his students and residents not to 'waste' their own educations by choosing work as 'useless' as I do."[19] I would add that the professor is not only cautioning these specific student physicians. He is upholding, first, the modernist medical project of attending to what is fixable and leaving the rest to unspecified others. Second, the professor asserts certain boundaries of the social body: those who are and are not worthy of medical expertise. Finally, the professor echoes the school boy who told Primo Levi how he could have escaped. The professor cannot accept that the chaos Hilfiker describes does not leave any way out.

The truth of the chaotic body is to reveal the hubris of other stories. Chaos stories show how quickly the props that other stories depend on can be kicked away. The limitation is that chaos is no way to live. Frederick Franck writes with his usual wisdom, "Poverty may be quite compatible with a religious attitude toward existence; destitution, hunger, utter humiliation negate it."[20] Among recent medical authors, none are able to look as long and as steadily at the dehumanizing effects of poverty as David Hilfiker. In the lives of those living in extreme poverty, illness cannot be other than chaos.

The unquestionable achievement of modernity was its emphasis on fixing: modernity requires faith to be accountable to what was being accomplished here on earth, in the conditions of people's everyday lives. The cost of modernity is to leave no place for people like Nancy, whose troubles are too complex, in both medical and social terms, for fixing. Sacks's orthopedic surgeon simply cannot hear his complaint that he feels his leg is not part of his body.

For those who share Hilfiker's and Franck's religious attitudes, the mystery of the chaos narrative is its opening to faith: "Blessed are the poor in spirit, for theirs is the kingdom of heaven" (Matthew 5:3). The greatest chaos stories are the first despairing verses of many of the Psalms; the Psalms' message seems to be that the redemption of faith can begin only in chaos. Tragically, those who are most destitute are often beyond such solace. For the poor in spirit to recognize their blessedness, some reflective space is required, and that reflection is what poverty, like unremitting pain, denies.

Six

The Quest Narrative

ILLNESS AND THE COMMUNICATIVE BODY

Restitution stories attempt to outdistance mortality by rendering illness transitory. Chaos stories are sucked into the undertow of illness and the disasters that attend it. Quest stories meet suffering head on; they accept illness and seek to *use* it. Illness is the occasion of a journey that becomes a quest. What is quested for may never be wholly clear, but the quest is defined by the ill person's belief that something is to be gained through the experience.

The quest narrative affords the ill person a voice as teller of her own story, because only in quest stories does the *teller* have a story to tell. In the restitution narrative the active player is the remedy: either the drug itself—as in the old advertisements where the drugs appeared as cartoon characters, charging around in the body—or the physician. Restitution stories are about the triumph of medicine; they are self-stories only by default. Chaos stories remain the sufferer's own story, but the suffering is too great for a self to be told. The voice of the teller has been lost as a result of the chaos, and this loss then perpetuates that chaos. Though both restitution and chaos remain background voices when the quest is foreground, the quest narrative speaks from the ill person's perspective and holds chaos at bay.

The quest narrative affords the ill their most distinctive voice, and most published illness stories are quest stories. Publication requires sustaining one's voice for a longer duration than oral stories require, some oral stories being as brief as a single remark. Yet only a few quest stories are published. Although this chapter concentrates on published quest stories, these represent a small fraction of what can be called the *enacted stories* of people's lives: involvement in patient advocacy is one enactment of a quest story; making significant vocational and personal changes in one's life following illness is another. By learning to hear the quest in published stories, appreciation of these enacted stories can be enhanced.

ILLNESS AS JOURNEY

The quest narrative certainly goes back to John Donne, who recast his critical illness, probably typhus, into a spiritual journey.[1] My nominee for parenthood for the contemporary quest story, however, is Friedrich Nietzsche. Nietzsche suffered from undiagnosed chronic ailments, including debilitating headaches. He wrote, "I have given a name to my pain, and call it 'dog.'" Nietzsche describes his pain as having the dog-like attributes of being faithful, obtrusive, shameless, entertaining, and clever. "I can scold it and vent my bad mood on it, as others do with their dogs, servants, and wives."[2]

I read this passage remembering that a threshold event in Nietzsche's final madness was his attempt to rescue a horse that was being beaten by its owner. The ironic truth of his illness description—if bad moods are to be vented, best to vent them on one's pain—conceals a moral commitment. Nietzsche anticipates what David Morris calls a "postmodern vision [that] would undermine a sense that we are slaves to pain (or even occasionally masters) by encouraging alternative ways of thinking."[3] Nietzsche calls his pain "dog" to jar the reader into a new relationship to illness. It seems a short step from Nietzsche to Anatole Broyard a century later, writing that "nobody wants an anonymous illness," and recommending that patients feel they have "earned" their illnesses.[4]

Quest stories tell of searching for alternative ways of being ill. As the ill person gradually realizes a sense of purpose, the idea that illness has been a journey emerges. The meaning of the journey emerges recursively: the journey is taken in order to find out what sort of journey one has been taking.

The narrative structure of this journey is best described by Joseph Campbell in his classic work, *The Hero With a Thousand Faces*.[5] I cite Campbell because of his preeminent influence on the popular culture of self-help and self-reflection.[6] Campbell is a popular moral philosopher who, regardless of his own influences, scholarship, or private personality, has profoundly affected the narrative presuppositions that inform illness stories. I mean "profoundly" in terms of both the extent of influence and the quality of influence. If the idea of "journey" has become a New Age spice sprinkled indiscriminately to season almost any experience, pop psychology could have done worse. The journey may be a fad, but it nevertheless represents a form of reflexive monitoring.

Campbell's description of the hero's journey can be reduced to three stages. The first is *departure,* beginning with a call. In illness stories the call is the symptom: the lump, dizziness, cough, or other sign that the body is not as it should be. The call is often refused, because the hero, who has not yet become a hero,[7] knows how much suffering will be involved. In illness stories the refusal may be the ill person's denial of the symptom. A woman who had lymphoma told of waking up, seeing a large lump on her neck, deciding it must be a dream, and going back to bed.

Eventually the call can no longer be refused—symptoms are unmistakable, diagnoses are made—and what Campbell calls "the first threshold" is crossed. For the ill person this first threshold may be hospitalization and surgery that determines the extent of the illness. Crossing the threshold begins the second stage, *initiation.* Tellers of quest stories use the metaphor of initiation implicitly and explicitly. Among the latter, Sue Nathanson's story of recovery from an abortion and tubal ligation ends with her friends staging a feminist goddess ceremony for her. The book closes with one of the women saying "The ritual begins *now.*"[8]

Nathanson's story demonstrates the reflexive quality of journeys: she is being formally initiated into the experience that has already initiated her. As in T. S. Eliot's famous lines in "Four Quartets," she has returned to her beginning and is now prepared to know the place. In illness initiations, unlike tribal ones, only at the end of the initiation does the teller conceptualize what has been going on *as* an initiation, thus organizing the experience as coherent and meaningful.

Campbell calls initiation "the road of trials," easily identified in any illness story as the various sufferings that illness involves, not only physical but also emotional and social. This road leads through other stages, such as temptation and atonement, until the ending or "apotheosis." The quest narrative tells self-consciously of being transformed; undergoing transformation is a significant dimension of the storyteller's responsibility. The end of the journey brings what Campbell calls a "boon." Quest stories of illness imply that the teller has been given something by the experience, usually some insight that must be passed on to others.

The final stage is the *return.* The teller returns as one who is no longer ill but remains marked by illness, as Schweitzer wrote of those who "bear the mark of the brotherhood of pain." This marked person lives in a world she has traveled beyond, a status well described by Campbell's phrase "master of the two worlds." Gail, a woman who suffers chronic pain, expresses this mastery when she asserts, "We have access to different experiences, different knowledges."[9]

Campbell's schematic of departure, initiation, and return for the hero's journey works well to describe the narrative structure of quest stories.[10] The sticking point is the notion of *hero:* what sort of "heroes" do ill people take themselves to be? Illness stories include some number of "I conquered . . ." stories.[11] This "conquering" heroism is on the modernist side of the postmodern divide. Campbell's postmodern appeal follows what Morris says about Nietzsche: his hero discovers alternative ways to experience suffering.

For me as a member of the remission society, Campbell deserves his influence because of his moral insight that mythic heroism is evidenced not by force of arms but by *perseverance.* The paradigmatic hero is not some Hercules wrestling and slugging his way through opponents, but the Bodhisattva, the compassionate being who vows to return to earth to share her enlightenment with others.[12] What the myths are about is agony.[13] The hero's moral status derives from being initiated through agony to atonement: the realization of oneness of himself with the world, and oneness of the world with its principle of creation. Suffering is integral to this principle, and learning the integrity of suffering is central to the boon.

The problem of return is to convince others that this atonement is a boon. As Campbell notes with regret, "The significant form of the human agony is lost to view."[14] The return thus sets in place the ill person's responsibility, and problem, of being a witness.

THREE FACETS OF QUEST

The range of quest stories is broad enough to make further specification useful. Quest stories have at least three facets: memoir, manifesto, and automythology.

The *memoir* combines telling the illness story with telling other events in the writer's life. The illness memoir could also be described as an interrupted autobiography. Most of the authors are persons whose public status would make them candidates for formal autobiography writing, but illness has required what would have been written later to be done earlier: Stewart Alsop's and Gilda Radner's memoirs are motivated by imminent death, and William Styron is rumored to have written about his depression in order to squelch other rumors about what happened to him.[15] Still other illness memoirs are fragments of an autobiography that the author prefers, for whatever postmodern reasons, to write in such fragments. John Updike's story of how psoriasis affected his life is an example.[16]

Events are not told chronologically in these memoirs, nor is a life rehearsed in detail. Rather, present circumstances become occasions for the recollection of certain past events. The illness constantly interrupts the telling of the past life, although alternatively, memories of the past life interrupt the present illness.

The memoir is the gentlest style of quest story. Trials are not minimized, but they are told stoically, without flourish. No special insight is claimed at the end; the insight is rather the incorporation—a good pun in this case—of illness into the writer's life. In the many illness memoirs by "famous" people, the memoir returns a life that has been publicly known through words and images back to the body with its tumors and tremors. The public person's split between media image and experienced reality is always a subtext of these stories and sometimes an explicit topic. Gilda Radner describes her need to find a balance between "being funny, being Gilda Radner, and being someone going through cancer."[17]

The least gentle quest stories are *manifestos*. In these stories the truth that has been learned is prophetic, often carrying demands for social action. Writers of manifestos underscore the responsibility that attends even provisional return from illness. Society is suppressing a truth about suffering, and that truth must be told. These writers do not want to go back to a former state of health, which is often viewed as a naive illusion. They want to use suffering to move others forward with them.

The clearest prophetic voice is that of Audre Lorde. Lorde's anger at social secrecy and hypocrisy finds its focus in demands that she begin wearing a breast prosthesis after her mastectomy. When she visits her surgeon's office ten days after surgery, the nurse points out she is not wearing a prosthesis. The observation turns into a order: "Usually supportive and understanding, the nurse now looked at me urgently and disapprovingly." The nurse's bottom line is, "We really like you to wear something, at least when you come in. Otherwise it's bad for the morale of the office." Lorde describes this incident as "only the first such assault on my right to define and to claim my own body."[18]

The issue expands from claiming her own body to claiming visual recognition of other women who bear her mark of pain. She does not want to conceal her difference but to affirm it, "because I have lived it, and survived it, and wish to share that strength with other women" (61). Women's enemy is silence; if silence is to turn into action, "then the first step is that women with mastectomies must become visible to each other." The alternative is isolation, not just as a woman with one breast, but as a human being facing mortality. Only by displaying our common mortality can humans accept this mortality as common and cease to fear it. "Yet once I face death as a life process," Lorde writes, "what is there possibly left for me to fear? Who can ever really have power over me again?" (61).

Disability stories frequently combine the facets of memoir and manifesto. Irving Zola, who had polio as a child, writes a memoir of visiting a village in the Netherlands, Het Dorp, that was built entirely for the needs of the disabled.[19] At the time of the visit Zola was already a successful sociologist, and the visit was arranged through professional channels while he was on sabbatical nearby. Arriving at the village, Zola decides to live as one of the disabled members. In myths the hero is often stripped of worldly possessions and powers as she enters the underworld where the adventure begins. In Zola's case he leaves behind the braces he walks with—symbolic of his professional status—and puts himself in a wheel chair, becoming one of the Het Dorp residents. His journal of the days that follow is a progressive self-discovery of all that he has denied about the effect of disability on his identity.

Het Dorp is a model of technological convenience for the disabled, yet it continues to remind Zola of "emotional needs that seemed to have been taken away, or never granted." His recognition of these needs leads him to a conclusion that is a manifesto. He realizes, uncomfortably, that the last twenty years of his life represent "a continuing effort to reclaim what I had lost—the right to act sexy, get angry, be vulnerable, and have possibilities" (214). After detailing how these rights are denied to the disabled, what rationalizations are used to justify these denials, and what resistance might restore these rights, Zola concludes in a prophetic voice: "If we lived in a less healthist, capitalist, and hierarchical society, which spent less time finding ways to exclude and disenfranchise people and more time finding ways to include and enhance the potentialities of everyone, then there wouldn't have been so much for me to overcome" (235). The manifesto asserts that illness is a social issue, not simply a personal affliction. It witnesses how society has added to the physical problems that disease entails, and it calls for change, based on solidarity of the afflicted.[20]

A third facet can be called the *automythology*.[21] The predominant metaphor of the automythology is the Phoenix, reinventing itself from the ashes of the fire of its own body. William May uses the Phoenix metaphor to describe the totality of self-reinvention following massive trauma or catastrophic illness.

"One cannot talk simply of a new accessory here, a change of venue there," May writes. "If the patient revives after such events, he must reconstruct afresh, tap new power, and appropriate patterns that help define a new existence."[22] Automythology fashions the author as one who not only has survived but has been reborn. Like the manifesto, the automythology reaches out, but its language is more personal than political. Individual change, not social reform, is emphasized, with the author as an exemplar of this change. The automythologist may be an unwilling hero, but he is never an unwitting one.

Oliver Sacks's *A Leg to Stand On* is an automythology with a narrative structure that follows Campbell's quest almost moment by moment. Sacks is injured while hiking, when he encounters a bull on a mountain side, runs away, and trips. The bull appears suddenly, focuses all manner of fears in Sacks, and then just as suddenly disappears. The bull's disappearance renders Sacks's initiation curiously self-induced: the proximate cause of his injury is both objective and intrapsychic.

Sacks then descends through several levels of hospitalization, descends to deeper psychic depths after surgery when his leg seems no longer his, and returns across several thresholds of rehabilitation. Each of these levels poses not only a physical but a moral challenge. At each threshold Sacks must always find new resources. Each of these, like the music that helps him to walk again, is invariably something that was at hand but not attended to: the music was not a piece he particularly cared for or admired. Part of the lesson is learning to see the ordinary as already containing all the resources one needs.

At the end of this process, Sacks claims a new identity, and here is the purest voice of automythology: "My adventure was ending. But I knew that something momentous had happened, which would leave its mark, and alter me, decisively, from now on. A whole life, a whole universe, had been compressed into these weeks: a destiny of experience neither given to, nor desired by, most men; but one which, having happened, would refashion and direct me."[23] Sacks has become Campbell's master of two worlds: he has traversed the experiential universe, suffered what few others have or would want to, and now makes his return. The language of automythology is heavy with words like *momentous, decisively, universe,* and *destiny.*

Other languages can serve the same end. Broyard creates his automythology from his tap dancing lessons and dancing language. Broyard treats his ordeals with an off-handedness that places him above his fate. His myth is his lightness, but this lightness remains his alone. A more inclusive automythology than Broyard or Sacks, and perhaps the best known of all illness stories, is Norman Cousins.

Cousins's first best-seller was *Anatomy of an Illness.*[24] In 1964 he returns from a diplomatic mission to the Soviet Union with symptoms that develop into an acute inflammatory disease of the connective tissue. The diagnosis is obscure and debated, but the debilitating effects are clear. Cousins finds it difficult to move, he develops nodules, suffers from "gravel-like substances under the skin" (30), and finally his jaw is almost locked. He is told his disease is "progressive and incurable" (45). Cousins's descent is complete as he contemplates paralysis.

The story of his return, further mythologized as a made-for-television movie with Ed Asner as Cousins, describes Cousins's "own total involvement" in his recovery. Cousins checks himself out of the hospital and into a nearby hotel suite, rented for one-third the cost. He takes massive intravenous doses of ascorbic acid, which he has read affects collagen breakdown and helps rheumatoid arthritis patients. He does all this as part of a therapeutic alliance with his friend and physician, who believes that "his biggest job was to encourage to the fullest the patient's will to live and to mobilize all the natural resources of the body and mind to combat disease" (44). The mission that Cousins thus attributes to his physician is his own philosophy in a nutshell.

The final part of his self-treatment is humor: Cousins encourages his will to live and helps his body mobilize its natural resources by watching slapstick movies and reading joke books. The reliance on humor is the basis of the myth of Cousins as the man who laughs himself well. His own account is more complex, reflecting Cousins's sophistication as a lay reader of the medical literature, but automythology prevails over possible placebo effects. Cousins takes laughter's therapeutic effects seriously, these effects both supporting and supported by his refusal to "accept the verdict" offered by the specialists.

The end of his book's first chapter shows Cousins's project: he rewrites the philosophy he developed as a political journalist into individualist medical terms, creating the automythology of his own recovery. Cousins ends the chapter with William James's idea that "human beings tend to live too far within self-imposed limits." Cousins holds up his recovery as showing how anyone can step beyond these limits. At issue is not merely medical cure but enhancing "the natural drive of the human mind and body toward perfectibility and regeneration. Protecting and cherishing that natural drive may well represent the finest exercise of human freedom" (48).

Cousins's language may be quieter than Sacks's, but his automythology claims more. Cousins cures himself, and this cure becomes metonymic for concepts of *perfectibility, regeneration,* and ultimately *the finest exercise of human freedom.* Cousins presents his automythology as potentially inclusive— anyone can laugh, thus anyone can mobilize his body's natural resources—but the story could only be his. Few patients move their treatment into hotel suites, research their own diseases, forge alliances with physicians who support eccentric treatment plans, and, through all this, keep laughing. Not least of Cousins's appeal is that his genuine humility affords others their own vicarious enjoyment of his privileges.

Automythology turns the specific illness into a paradigm of universal conflicts and concerns. The body of the storyteller becomes a pivot point between microcosm and macrocosm, and human potential—"freedom" for Cousins and "destiny" for Sacks—depends on whether the lessons that the storyteller has learned can be accepted and practiced by others.

THE COMMUNICATIVE BODY

The communicative body is told in quest stories, but more importantly, quest stories are one ethical *practice* of this body.

The quest hero accepts *contingency* because the paradox learned on the quest is that surrendering the superficial control of health yields control of a higher order. Lorde expresses this paradox when she writes that only by facing death can she become someone over whom no one has power.[25]

The quest teaches that contingency is the only real certainty. If Lorde expresses this lesson in political terms, Madeleine L'Engle, writing of the time just after her husband died, expresses it as a spiritual truth. She describes her situation by quoting a bishop saying of his wife's death, "I have been all the way to the bottom. And it is solid."[26] The point of suffering, from a spiritual perspective, is that *only* the bottom is solid. L'Engle writes of her husband's illness, "We have had to be open to crisis" (181). Being open to crisis as a source of change and growth and valuing contingency even with its suffering are the bases of the communicative body.

The desire of this contingent body is *productive*, but the direction of this desire—unlike the desire of the mirroring body—is conditioned by its *dyadic* relation to others. In the Buddhist metaphor of the Bodhisattva, the communicative body desires to save all beings. Posthumous illness stories have a particularly Bodhisattva-like quality. Why does someone like Alsop or Radner or Broyard spend his or her last months of consciousness and energy writing about illness? These people had every other option of entertainment or companionship open to them, but they chose to write. Why does Lorde, immediately after her mastectomy, expend her energy writing? The tautological answer is that reaching out to others is what the dyadic body does; its desire is to touch others and perhaps to make a difference in the unfolding of their stories.

Writing is not, as it could be, a means of dissociation from one's own body. Quest storytellers write of their own bodies, including pains and disfigurements, in sensuous detail. Their *association* with their bodies allows them to feel Schweitzer's "mark of pain" upon their flesh and to see the pain in the other's flesh. Body association is the ground of dyadic relatedness, just as dyadic relatedness and desire are inseparable.

Seeking to be *for* the other, reaching out as a way of being, does not mean rescuing this other from his own contingency. What will happen to the other person, what he will end up suffering, remains as contingent as what happens to the self. Communicative bodies seek instead to affect how the other understands her embodied contingency. To use Campbell's terms, the communicative body seeks to share the boon that it has gained upon its own return. Others need this boon for the journeys they necessarily will undertake.

This boon, describable only in another tautology, is the body's ability to grasp itself reflectively as a communicative body: to *be* associated with itself, open to contingency, dyadic toward others, and desiring for itself in relation to others. The nature of this boon is that it must be shared, which means sharing the self. The story is one medium through which the communicative body recollects itself as having become what it *is*, and through the story the body offers itself to others. Recollection of self and self-offering are inseparable, each being possible only as the complement of the other.

QUEST AS SELF-STORY

In quest stories the interruption is reframed as a challenge. The self-story hinges on William May's question, "How did I rise to the occasion?" The genesis of the quest is some occasion requiring the person to be more than she has been, and the purpose is becoming one who has risen to that occasion. This occasion at first appears as an interruption but later comes to be understood as an opening.

A woman whom Deborah Kahane calls Terri expresses what is said in almost every quest story: "I would never have *chosen* to be taught this way but I like the changes in me. I guess I had to go to the edge to get there."[27] What started the illness is secondary to the effect of going "to the edge." Terri's purpose is coming back from that edge to become the person she is, someone who is changed. Illness was an interruption she would not have chosen, but she now accepts it as the cost of changes she likes. Losses continue to be mourned, but the emphasis is on gains.

The "changes" that ground Terri's statement are changes of character: *who* she is. Character merges both *persona,* the character in the story, and quality, having a good character. The self-story must go beyond simply claiming changes in character and demonstrate these changes. Much of the success of the story—its impact both on others and on the self—depends on how convincing this display of changed character is. Readers pick up published illness stories for all sorts of reasons, but the moral purpose of reading is *to witness a change of character through suffering.* In this witness the reader both affirms that change, which is one sort of moral duty, and gains a model for his own change, another moral duty.

The most extreme change is the automythological claim to have become someone else. Sacks claims to be altered, "decisively, from now on."[28] The essence of his alteration is that he is now prepared to discover what he calls, in his own emphasis, *"a neurology of the soul."* He now sees his way beyond his intellectual mentors and claims to have found "a new field . . . a new and true way of thinking" (222).

This latter statement constitutes a promissory note. In the redemption of this promise, *A Leg to Stand On* does not stand alone, and possibly could not stand alone. Most readers of *A Leg to Stand On* will read the book informed by who Sacks became: best-selling author, portrayed by Robin Williams in the movie version of Sacks's book, *Awakenings.* The promissory note at the end of *A Leg to Stand On* is thus read as substantially redeemed. Sacks's hyperbole about his new self and new neurology, which could fall flat if he were otherwise unknown, is forceful. Sacks really *has* produced a new "neurology of the soul." But the automythology of his illness story requires his other stories to make fully credible the change of character he claims.

Most stories tell of less dramatic changes. What tellers discover is not someone wholly new, but rather "who I always have been."[29] This self is not so newly discovered as newly *connected* to its own memory. The past is reinterpreted in terms of the present and takes on an enhanced meaning. This present is no longer a contingent graft on a past that was supposed to lead elsewhere.

Audre Lorde establishes this newly connected self when she asks the rhetorical question, "How did the Amazons of Dahomey feel?"—referring to Amazon warriors whose initiation involved having one breast cut off, the better to shoot a bow.[30] Lorde thus fashions a potent metaphor for her new identity, the one-breasted woman warrior, complete with third-world location and lesbian connotations. This metaphor joins her post-mastectomy body to her earlier black, lesbian, feminist self. The power of the metaphor is to give the mastectomy a kind of retrospective necessity: she had to lose a breast to become the full version of what she was before, but then only incompletely. Her metaphor becomes what Schafer (chapter 3, above) calls the storyline of her self-story.

Lorde's rhetorical question about the Amazons of Dahomey convinces readers of her self-change because this change is *not* new but represents a recollection. Lorde has become what she always has been, but empowered by the full knowledge and the now embodied scars of that identity. The metaphor of the Dahomey Amazon is the epiphany of Lorde's becoming; it expresses her character because coming up with the metaphor—telling it—is the expression of her character.

Self-change seems remarkably unrelated to gender, and a story similar to Lorde's is told by Robert Murphy, whose demographic profile is as unlike Lorde's as could be found. Murphy was a prominent academic anthropologist, chair of his department at Columbia, when he noticed symptoms that were eventually diagnosed as a benign tumor in his spine. The growth of this tumor eventually renders him quadriplegic. His illness story juxtaposes his body's deterioration and restriction with his mind's expansion. Murphy compares illness to an anthropological field trip and finds the medical worlds he enters "no less strange" than the jungles he traveled in to do research.[31]

From his research Murphy finds the metaphor that joins who he has become with who he always has been. As he writes his book he is almost totally paralyzed, strapped in a chair, moving only his fingers over the keyboard of his computer. He writes, "My narration bears an eerie resemblance to the myth-telling of the shamans of the . . . Peruvian Amazon, who . . . relate their myths while holding their bodies absolutely motionless" (222). Not just the credibility but the morality of Murphy's change lies in this metaphorical joining of his past to his present. No promissory note is offered here: the metaphor itself delivers what it promises.

Murphy, on his own description, would not fit the ideal type of the communicative body. He describes himself dealing with his physical degeneration by "radical dissociation" from his body. This dissociation is made easier because he "never did take much pride in my body. . . . I cultivated my wits instead" (101). I can hardly disagree with Murphy's self-description, but I can argue that in his telling he is associated with his body. In the shaman metaphor, Murphy's body is not only the subject of his telling but, in its rigidity, the medium of this telling. Just as the shamans' telling somehow depends on how they hold their bodies, so Murphy's telling does also. Earlier in his life Murphy may not have taken much pride in his body, but as he writes he places enormous metaphorical, and even mythic, weight upon it.

Murphy's story works because his body sustains its weight, just as Lorde's life and Sacks's writings sustain what is claimed through their bodies. As storytellers of their illnesses, each more than rises to the occasion. Character is demonstrated, reflexively, in the writing that is the measuring up of that character.

Realizing who they always have been, truly been, each becomes or prepares to become the re-created, moral version of that self. In this display of character, memory is revised, interruption assimilated, and purpose grasped. "Whatever has happened to me or will happen," the storyteller as hero implicitly claims, "the purpose remains mine to determine."

Three Ethics of Self-Story

Because the communicative body is dyadic, the self-story is never just a *self*-story but becomes a self/*other*-story. In telling

voice
memory
responsibility

such a story, the three issues of voice, memory, and responsibility merge. Finding a voice becomes the problem of taking responsibility for memory. Different quest stories all express this voice-memory-responsibility intersection. The self-story thus becomes an ethical practice of the communicative body. Three ethics, as overlapping as the three styles of quest, suggest the diversity of responsibility in storytelling.

An *ethic of recollection* is practiced when one who recollects shares memories of past action. Displaying one's past to others requires taking responsibility for what was done. Past actions can be disapproved, but they cannot be disowned; no one else did them, and they cannot be changed. The story is a moral opportunity to set right what was done wrong or incompletely.

When Audre Lorde was told to wear a prosthesis, she reports being "too outraged to speak then."[32] The key word is *then*. Human frailty is such that *then*, at the time of the outrage or impasse or whatever dilemma, voice may fail. Lorde's ethical action lies in her willingness to recollect that failure and offer it to others with an indication of what should have been done. She may have lapsed *then*, but she uses her outrage to speak more clearly and to many more people in her recollected story. The voice she finds fulfills her responsibility to memory.

An *ethic of solidarity and commitment* is expressed when the storyteller offers his voice to others, not to speak for them, but to speak *with* them as a fellow-sufferer who, for whatever reasons of talent or opportunity, has a chance to speak while others do not. When Zola takes off the leg braces that allow him to walk upright, he expresses solidarity with Het Dorp residents confined to wheel chairs. As he finds the wheel chair suits his body better in some ways, he gains the prophetic voice to express all that sustaining appearances of "normality" cost him and other disabled persons. The manifesto expressing such a prophetic voice becomes a kind of rallying point, which is how many women with cancer use Lorde's book.

Finally, quest stories practice an *ethic of inspiration*. Humans need exemplars who inspire. The heroic stance of the automythologist inspires because it is rooted in woundedness; the agony is not concealed. Sacks tells how despondent he was after his surgery. Cousins details the nearly complete incapacity of his body when his symptoms were most intense. Their stories show what is possible in impossible situations, and thus point toward what Cousins calls freedom.

These three ethics—recollection, solidarity, inspiration—overlap, just as memoir, prophetic voice, and automythology overlap in any story. Both the styles of quest story and their respective ethics are facets of the communicative body. They are practices this body adopts variously, as contingent situations require.

The quest self-story is about voice finding itself: when the nurse tells Audre Lorde to wear a prosthesis, Lorde is rendered speechless for a moment; from this she learns the awful potential of silence. The problem of being seriously ill becomes the problem of finding a voice. Lorde writes, "I was going to die, if not sooner then later, whether or not I had ever spoken myself. My silences had not protected me. Your silence will not protect you."[33]

Voice is found in the recollection of memories. The storyteller's responsibility is to witness the memory of what happened, and to set this memory right by providing a better example for others to follow. Lorde summarizes this responsibility as it only can be summarized, in the most particularistic terms, because each of us can only witness from the particularity of who we are: "Because I am woman, because I am black, because I am a lesbian, because I am myself, a black woman warrior poet doing my work, come to ask you, are you doing yours?" (21). Taking up this challenge is the ethical practice of the self-story.

FROM QUEST TO TESTIMONY

The quest narrative recognizes ill people as responsible moral agents whose primary action is witness; its stories are necessary to restore the moral agency that other stories sacrifice.

Ill people need to be regarded by themselves, by their caregivers, and by our culture as heroes of their own stories. Modernism made the physician, specifically the surgeon, into the hero of illness. In this modernist construction, heroism is not perseverance but *doing*. Ill people's passive heroism, when recognized in obituaries, is equated with a stoicism that is praised for its silence. Quest stories as they are told, and chaos stories when they are honored, call for a shift from the hero as Hercules to the hero as Bodhisattva; from the hero of force to the hero of perseverance through suffering. The story is the means for perseverance to become active, reaching out to others, asserting its own ethic.

This shift in heroic style challenges fundamental presuppositions of modernity. The modernist hero is a person of action and, as Bauman observes, of abstract ideals. For such a hero, conquering illness is itself a cause, and a cause that may supersede the immediate welfare of the particular ill person.[34] The wounded hero of illness stories speaks only of what she has experienced. In offering a personal experience to another person, the hero of illness quests is more like Bauman's postmodern moral person, oriented to "the life or well-being or dignity of another human being."[35]

The problem for storytellers who would be moral persons is keeping in mind what Paul Ricoeur writes about prophetic testimony: the prophet receives his testimony from elsewhere.[36] The opportunity to tell one's own illness story as one wants to tell it—in one's "own" voice—is a kind of grace. Campbell is always clear that undertaking the hero's journey requires grace; the hero who thinks he travels on his own will fail.

Falling into the hubris that one's voice can ever be entirely one's own is only one of the failures that quest stories risk. Automythologies can easily become stories to reassure the healthy that just as the author has risen above illness, they too can escape. The antidote to this pretense of invulnerability is chaos stories, reminding us that some situations cannot be risen above. Most significantly, quest stories risk romanticizing illness. Here the antidote is restitution stories, reminding us that any sane person would rather be healthy, and most of us need the help of others to sustain that health.

The risk of quest stories is like the risk of the Phoenix metaphor: they can present the burning process as too clean and the transformation as too complete, and they can implicitly deprecate those who fail to rise out of their own ashes. Many ill people invoke the Phoenix to describe their experiences, but May expresses a significant reservation about this metaphor. While the Phoenix remembers nothing of its former life, the victim of some trauma—May writes specifically of burn victims here—does remember.[37] May's reservation is given added force by Lawrence Langer writing on Holocaust witnesses.

Langer quotes the Auschwitz memoirs of Charlotte Delbo, who "uses the image of a serpent shedding its own skin and emerging with a 'fresh and shining' one."[38] The problem is that renewal is never complete: "She knows that though shedding a skin may leave the snake unchanged, similar results apply to *her* only in appearance" (4).

Ultimately, her experience is too complex for the serpent metaphor, and probably for any metaphor: "The skin covering the memory of Auschwitz is tough," Delbo writes. "Sometimes, however, it bursts, and gives back its contents." She tells how her embodied memories of Auschwitz came back to re-possess her in a dream. She feels herself "pierced with cold, filthy, gaunt, and the pain is so unbearable, so exactly the pain I suffered there, that I feel it again physically, I feel it again through my whole body" (6–7).

Delbo upsets the Phoenix metaphor, showing it to be too clean, too heroic. After reading Delbo I hear the Phoenix storyline as a restitution narrative that conceals the agony. I myself am no Phoenix. Whenever one of my own medical tests requires "further investigation," the skin that covers over the memories of my first cancer bursts. I do not suggest my experience has anything of the terror of Delbo's, but suddenly the pain of having cancer bears down on me again with all its indescribable weight. Each time I learn how close to the surface those memories remain.

Metaphors, as Lorde and Murphy show, can be powerful means to healing. But generalized metaphors, offered as storylines for others' self-stories, are dangerous. The Phoenix does not mourn what lies in its ashes; the serpent does not mourn its old skin. Human illness, even when lived as a quest, always returns to mourning. The boon is gaining the ability to mourn not for oneself only, but for others.

Seven   *Testimony*

I once spoke at a conference for persons who had cancer or
were in remission. One of the organizers opened the conference by posing the question of what we—he himself was currently in treatment—should call ourselves. He proposed
"survivors," dating one's survival from the time of diagnosis. I
have no quarrel with the notion of survivors, but my first choice
as a designation is "witness."

Survival does not include any particular responsibility other
than continuing to survive. Becoming a witness assumes a responsibility for telling what happened. The witness offers testimony to a truth that is generally unrecognized or suppressed.
People who tell stories of illness are witnesses, turning illness
into moral responsibility.

Bringing back the "boon" at the end of the quest narrative is
self-concious testimony. The chaos narrative requires a listener who is prepared to hear it as testimony; Nancy's im-
mersion in her frenzied telling of her multiple interruptions
(chapter 5) prevents her from hearing herself as a witness. The
restitution narrative is the least obvious form of testimony, but
it too tells a truth: the will to live, to cure and be cured.

The postmodern affinity for testimony is one response—
and often a frustrated one—to the accumulated chaos stories
of modernity; testimony tells these stories.[1] Thus testimony,
for all its commitment to truth and its ability to break through

the limits of what its times attend to, is itself another construction of its times. The more that is told, the more we are made conscious of remaining on the edge of a silence. How much remains that can never be told is unknown.

But to observe that testimony is incomplete and only possible at a particular cultural moment in no way diminishes the force of that testimony. To paraphrase the quotation from William James that orients this whole inquiry, no analysis can ever "settle the hash" of testimony. Any analysis is always left gazing at what remains in excess of the analyzable. What is testified to remains the really real, and in the end what counts are duties toward it.

POSTMODERN TESTIMONY

Shoshana Felman describes testimony as "composed of bits and pieces of a memory that has been overwhelmed by occurrences that have not settled into understanding or remembrance, acts that cannot be constructed as knowledge nor assimilated into full cognition, events in excess of our frames of reference."[2] The sentence's repeated "that" phrases seem to chase what can never quite be said; Felman's own language seems overwhelmed, especially as I read it aloud. Testimony has that effect: it overwhelms even as it is overwhelmed.

Felman's description evokes what is postmodern in contemporary testimony: even as "truth" is told, we now find uncertainty. Even in testimony, consciousness struggles to gain sovereignty over its own experience. Felman's book is one example of current academic interest in testimony; books like Art Spiegelman's *Maus I* and *II*[3] and films like *Schindler's List* exemplify the popular culture of testimony. But as a form of testimony, the proliferation of Holocaust materials is dwarfed by the self-help movement with its various forms of "recovery."

Recovery, with its paradigm form in the Alcoholics Anonymous Twelve Step Program, is based on the popular availability of testimony as a commonsense activity. The different facets of this movement then reinforce the cultural importance of testimony. Published illness stories ride this wave of interest in testimony.

Each of these testimonies presents itself as some fragment of a larger whole that the individual witness makes no pretense of grasping in its entirety. Postmodern testimony speaks not in what Jean-François Lyotard called "grand narratives"[4]—the narratives of church, state, science, and medicine that held earlier societies and lives together; rather, it speaks in Felman's bits and pieces. These bits and pieces are all that an "overwhelmed" consciousness can deal with. A grand narrative is the work of a sovereign consciousness that claims the ability to assimilate experience into what Felman calls "full cognition." This sovereignty depends on experiences fitting into existing frames of reference.

Consciousness loses its sovereignty when the frames of reference that once could assimilate experience have been hauled across the postmodern divide. In postmodern times, events now happen, and are acknowledged to happen, in excess of those frames. This excess takes at least two forms: too many events happen too fast to be fitted into appropriate frames, and some events simply do not fit even when reflective space is available for the fitting. As both forms of excess act together, the old frames no longer contain the pace and breadth of new experiences.

At the root of the overwhelmed memory that Felman finds in testimony is a *body* that is overwhelmed. Audre Lorde hears the nurse's order to wear a prosthesis as threatening "my right to define and to claim my own body." Her body—what it means to define and to claim it—is the point of contest in her testimony. As she writes of her body, Lorde is caught in the same expressive dilemma that Felman, or I, or anyone else shares. "Define" and even "claim" are still too verbal, too cognitive: the body is the excess of any definitions or stated claims; it is in excess of any language that testimony can speak. What Felman calls "full cognition," the ideal of a consciousness that can be sovereign over its experiences, seems impossible. The body is always "more," which is why desire is always an issue. Bodies want "more," because the body *is* "more."

What, then, can be said about the testimony of the ill, since this testimony is already an excess of what can be spoken? The post-colonial, embodied self pushes the limits of testimony.

The Body's Testimony

The witness in a traffic court speaks on the authority of having been there, on the scene; what counts is seeing. The illness witness also speaks from having being there, but his testimony is less of seeing and more of *being*. Gabriel Marcel expresses this quality of witness: "We are concerned with a certainty which I *am* rather than with a certainty which I have." This certainty is realized in testimony: "But how can I *be* a certainty," Marcel asks, "if not in as much as I am a living testimony?"[5]

Marcel's notion of being a living testimony focuses the quality of witness offered by illness stories and further explains how illness stories are not only *about* the body but *of* and through the body. The content that illness stories offer is valuable for a variety of purposes: for the teller's reordering of her life story, as guidance to others who will follow, and to provide caregivers with an understanding of what the ill experience. But the body testifies in excess of all these contents.

Illness stories are told by bodies that are themselves the living testimony; the proof of this testimony is that the witnesses *are* what they testify. Others can *have* the story as content, just as throughout this book I have many stories and retell them. But only the ill person herself can *be* the story, and that being—the excess of any content—is the plenitude of testimony and its demand.

In the previous chapter I quoted a woman called Gail who suffers from chronic pain. Gail's comments, as recorded by Linda Garro, are some of the finest testimony available, while also raising questions of what this testimony is. Gail refers to "people who don't have pain" as "normals," and to "the medical establishment" as "whitecoats":

> And all these people in pain . . . all these people with aches and all these people suffering. We walk in different dimensions. We have access to different experiences, different knowledges. And there are so many of us, too. What would happen if we all knew what it really meant and we all lived as if it really mattered, which it does. We could help the normals and the whitecoats both. We could help them see that they're wasting the precious moments of their lives, if they would look at us who don't have it. I'm convinced only sick people know what health is. And they know it by its very loss.[6]

Gail claims different knowledges, but what would her answer be if she were called to account for such knowledge? What if a group of professionals were to examine her and ask, *what exactly* do you have to teach?

Gail could certainly say this and that about delivery of health care, but her true witness, the witness that "really matters" to use her phrase, is not what she could say but what she *is*. Available language forces Gail to speak of what she is in terms of knowledge, but her "knowledge" is in excess of speech. Her knowledge comes down to this: living as if it really mattered, which it does, and not wasting precious moments. Everyone knows these things, but Gail, through her years of pain, *knows* them.

Gail wants normals and whitecoats to *look* at her; the necessity to choose one verb limits her, but her choice is important. For testimony in traffic court a written deposition will suffice. The witness of suffering must be *seen* as a whole body, because embodiment is the essence of witness. Gail's knowledge and the difference it could make emanate from the site of her pain, which is the source of this knowledge. Her testimony is her body, and ultimately the body can only be apprehended through all the senses of another body.

A witness such as Gail cannot be *asked* what her testimony is; asking is the least dimension of her demand to be witnessed. Those who would receive Gail's testimony must receive her, because she *is* that testimony. Thus the witness makes a witness of others; a particular quality of the word witness is its movement of outward concentric circles. When someone receives the testimony of another, that person becomes a witness, and so on.

Art Spiegelman's *Maus I* and *II* exemplify this concentric quality. The books' subtitle, "A Survivor's Tale," refers ambiguously both to Vladek Spiegelman, Art's father and a survivor of Auschwitz, and to Art himself, who survives his mother's suicide and a childhood haunted by comparisons to an older brother who died in the Holocaust. The books tell Art's struggle to survive his father's memories. *Maus I* and *II* are as much about the effect of the Holocaust on children of survivors as on the survivors themselves. The books' effect on the next circle of witnesses, the readers, is left open.

One message of Art's survival is that none of us can be detached spectators to others' witness. He comes to terms with his father by eliciting his testimony, recording it, interpreting it, and ultimately presenting it to a broader audience of witnesses. The imperative to receive testimony is postmodern but not distinctively so; the distinctive postmodernism lies in the witness's uncertainty of what is being received. Art remains profoundly ambivalent about his father. Even as he honors his father's testimony, he recognizes his father's less attractive behaviors and questions whether these can be excused as results of wartime trauma. However he attempts to sort out the levels of testimony and responsibility, consciousness will never be sovereign over experience. What is certain is his own inescapable place in the circle of testimony. Testimony is distinct from other reports because it does not simply affect those who receive it; testimony *implicates* others in what they witness.

This reciprocity of witnessing requires not one communicative body but a *relationship of* communicative bodies. Ordinary speech, conditioned by thinking on the model of law courts, refers to "the witness" as if witnessing could be a solitary act. Witnessing always implies a relationship; I tell myself stories all the time, but I cannot testify to myself alone. Part of what turns stories into testimony is the call made upon another person to receive that testimony. Testimony calls on its witnesses to become what none of us are yet, communicative bodies. When Vladek and Art share the testimony of the Holocaust, as survivor and artist respectively, they communicate, and may have their only moments of communion with each other.

In its testimony the communicative body calls others into a dyadic relationship. Testimony as an activity defines the communicative body, albeit tautologically and recursively. Gail becomes a witness to her illness because she is a communicative body, but she also becomes a communicative body through her testimony. The communicative body jumps out of its isolating compartment in my too neat diagram in chapter 2 and requires another body. The dominating body also jumps out of its slot, because it needs the subservience of the other in order to be.

The communicative body needs the other in order to commune.

Testimony like Gail's cannot be called to account because that mode of interrogation isolates her: for others to require her to give them an analytical specification of her "knowledge" is already to destroy the being that is the basis of that knowledge, which is Gail's communicative body. Living like it really matters, which it does, is living in communion with others. The excess of this communion over any verbal account is suggested by Jodi Halpern, defining empathic care as "attuned . . . through preverbal resonance."[7] The only appropriate response to Gail is not, "What do you have to tell me?" but rather, "Let me be with you." The only mode for receiving testimony such as hers is *being with*.

The content of illness stories, the events, actions and responses they tell, are openings to their more fundamental testimony, which is the *presence* of the embodied teller. Illness stories require an interplay of mutual presences: the listener must be present as a potentially suffering body to receive the testimony that is the suffering body of the teller. This presupposition of embodied presence could not be further from the practice of literary deconstruction, with its negation of the author's presence and treatment of the story as "text."[8]

Yet to understand illness stories as testimony is to use them in a deconstructive way. They disassemble what Dorothy Smith calls the "relations of ruling" inherent in the administrative texts—medical charts, financial statements, hospital administrative procedures—that mediate the lives of ill people.[9] The testimony of the illness story asserts the embodied presence that these administrative texts simultaneously rely on and deny, like the colonial texts described by Spivak (see chapter 1). The body of the ill person is the reason medical administration exists, but medicine as scientific, professional activity can only recognize the body as carrier of the disease. The experience of embodiment eludes official medical discourse, however attuned many practicing physicians are to their patients' experiences.[10]

The change that testimony like Gail's calls for is not some reorganization of "service delivery" or enhanced "communication skills" among physicians. The issue is nothing less than changing the cultural milieu so that people like Gail are *seen* for what their bodies testify to. The demand of her testimony is for other bodies to *commune* with her in her pain, because only through her pain has she learned what really matters. Normals and whitecoats can learn what really matters only through communion with her; in that communion they can stop wasting precious moments. This communion takes place outside the language of survival, which it thus challenges. Communion is not instrumental and not conditional, and so administrative systems have no place for it.

Testifying to illness as a communicative body may be an individual moral choice, but this testimony implies a social ethic.

THE PEDAGOGY OF SUFFERING

Testimony is complete in itself, but it requires commentary in order to be transformed into a social ethic. Gail's testimony, quoted above, is that the ill offer others a truth. The "pedagogy of suffering" is the phrase I have used in my own earlier writing to describe what the ill have to teach society.

By conceiving suffering as a pedagogy, agency is restored to ill people; testimony is given equal place alongside professional expertise. The pedagogy of suffering does not replace modernist medicine and supporting theories such as the sick role; rather what is opened is the possibility for shifting between frameworks as required by *responding* to the ill. The sick role is useful not only as a lightning rod for criticism of modernist medicine; it retains much explanatory force. The restitution story remains the most frequently told of illness narratives, and modernist medicine thrives: most discontents are demands for more medicine.

But times change. Modernist medicine has regarded suffering as a puzzle to be "controlled" if not eradicated. Postmodern illness culture, lay and medical, recognizes a need to accept suffering as an intractable part of the human condition.[11] I understand postmodernity as a period of frameworks shifting in and out of foreground and background. Donald Levine has recommended that social theory become "multivocal."[12] Clinical ethics and concepts of care must also become multivocal.

Society needs a pedagogy of suffering. The finest defender of modernity, Jürgen Habermas, also delineates most clearly its dark side: the processes he calls the colonization of everyday, communal lifeworlds of human bodies by administrative systems that are driven by demands for profits and votes.[13] The postmodernity I want to defend is not so different from Habermas's modernity: where he foregrounds the continuing relevance of the modernist project while recognizing problems that require change, I foreground change while recognizing continuities.

The pedagogy of suffering is my antidote to administrative systems that cannot take suffering into account because they are abstracted from the needs of bodies. When the body's vulnerability and pain are kept in the foreground, a new social ethic is required.

The challenge is to state this ethic in terms that remain multivocal. A multivocal ethic does not imply relativism; it suggests the recognition of difference that seems to be the original impetus behind Habermas's work: the need to recognize multiple voices and afford each full legitimacy in reaching a consensus that is not only workable in achieving minimal compliance of all parties, but is also moral in the sense of respecting the values of all whose compliance is required.

The need for a new, multivocal clinical ethic is starkly demonstrated in a quotation reported by Charles Bosk in his research on physicians who are genetic counselors. Bosk asks one of the physicians he has been working with and studying how he "came to grips with all the 'accidents' or 'mistakes' [of medical practice] that he saw." The response should be read aloud to every medical school class as an example of how professional practice can warp an otherwise decent mind:

> What you have to do is this, Bosk. When you get up in
> the morning, pretend your car is a spaceship. Tell
> yourself you are going to visit another planet. You say,
> "On that planet terrible things happen, but they don't
> happen on my planet. They only happen on that
> planet I take my spaceship to each morning."[14]

Robert Zussman suggests the same attitude when he summarizes his research on intensive care units by saying the staff "live in a moral universe of limited liability."[15]

Zussman defends this attitude, at least to some extent. He points out, correctly, that "the impersonality of medicine" and the "disappearance of an orientation to the patient as a person" are the price paid for "the disappearance of a sometimes oppressive moralizing" (29). The limitation of liability at least cuts both ways: drug dealers and patients whose conditions result from their own bad habits get the same care as anyone else, or at least they do in Zussman's observations.[16]

Bosk provides the epigram for what I would call "spaceship ethics," and Zussman adds a reminder that even indifference can have its benefits. What is required in clinical ethics is not a replacement of existing orientations but their displacement within a multivocality that recognizes the respective legitimacies of various claims and finds ways to balance these claims, making each aware of the others. In a multivocal medical world, non-medical voices would be heard. Physicians would take responsibility for their part in creating the "other planet," and others would recognize that physicians do not create the world of medicine exactly as they choose.

The practice of clinical ethics struggles to harmonize a rapidly changing medical practice, pushed in new directions by administrative, technological, and cultural changes, with the older modernist assumptions of professional expertise, administrative rationalization, and the possessive individualism of a capitalist system. I intend no irony in writing that these modernist assumptions are supported by real payoffs: I was lucky to have testicular cancer at the older end of the disease's age range; if I had had it at the younger end, the drugs that treated me successfully would not yet have been in general use.

The payoffs are real, but the tragedies incurred by spaceship ethics are equally real, and popular awareness of the tragic potential in medical treatment grows. The "choice-in-dying" movement is one social indicator of distrust in end-of-life medical care; another is women's discontents and health activism on issues ranging from hysterectomy rates to the safety of breast implants.[17] The problem is that as long as clinical ethics remains grounded in the assumptions of modernity, it is unable to offer an adequate response to such distrust and discontent; as long as limited liability remains the guiding principle governing its vision of the practice of medicine, clinical ethics limits itself to imagining variations in limitation on liability. It keeps on shuffling the same deck.

Nancy Mairs, whose years with multiple sclerosis have given her time to contemplate relationships of mutual giving, proposes a radically different ethic of *extensive responsibility*. Mairs observes that charity "is never nice."[18] People who give in order to be nice do not think of themselves as needy; the needy are others. To be harsher than Mairs is, the "nice" need the needy to be other to their niceness, but—returning to Spivak's argument (see chapter 1) about master texts—the nice cannot acknowledge their need for the needy. Thus charity turns into domination: the nice make the needy dependent upon them.

The relations of giving that Mairs imagines begin in a *mutual* recognition of need. Mairs's counterintuitive insight is that *all* persons have abundances, and all have lacks: "True, your abundance may complement someone else's lack, which you are moved to fill, but since your lacks are being similarly filled, perhaps by the same person, perhaps by another, reciprocity rather than domination frames the interchanges" (163). Mairs certainly knows that these abundances "may not take a form you much like" (163), such as multiple sclerosis for her or cancer for her husband. Too often one's abundance is suffering. But the recognition of suffering as abundance is one pillar of a charity that is not domination but reciprocity.

The other pillar is Mairs's faith that each person is lacking. Her argument finds a complement in David Hilfiker's explanation of why he took up the practice of poverty medicine, with the loss of income, comfort, and prestige that move entailed. Poverty medicine is an antidote to his own "brokenness."[19] Seeing oneself as "broken" goes against the current of contemporary North American culture, particularly professional culture. The reorientation Mairs proposes is radical. When a person believes, truly, in her own lack, then filling that lack is a matter of need. "Charity" becomes a way of meeting one's own need by drawing on the abundance of others, which happens to be an abundance of need.

Again, this need is certainly not an abundance that the needy want, nor does it make the needy attractive; quite the contrary. Mairs has spent enough time among the destitute to have lost any illusions about the effects of poverty, and Hilfiker struggles constantly with his lack of sympathy for many of his patients. It is precisely the unsympathetic aspect of the needy that makes filling their need into a remedy for brokenness.

Genuine service, for Mairs and Hilfiker, is a matter not of being nice but of recognizing that one's own lack can only be met by the other's abundance of need. Applied to medicine, this thinking displaces Parsons's idea of the physician acting as social control agent to regulate abuses of the privileges supposedly afforded the ill. Instead, what emerges is an image of the physician as servant who understands himself as being served: Jesus washing the feet of his disciples is the appropriate ideal. The paradox that as we serve we are also being served is the core of Mairs's ethic; our deepest human needs can *only* be served in relations created by our service.

If people could believe that each of us lacks something that only an other can fill—if we could be communicative bodies—then empathy would no longer be spoken of as something one person "has for" another. Instead, empathy is what a person "is with" another: a relationship in which each understands herself as requiring completion by the other.[20] The ill person is then no longer the passive patient imagined by the sick role, who receives care against the promise of returning to productive work. The sick-role conception places care within the language of survival: caring is rendered instrumental and contingent.

The pedagogy of suffering means that one who suffers has something to teach, just as Gail claims, and thus has something to give, as Mairs recognizes. Relationships of caring are no longer asymmetrical, even though the real instrumental *work* of doing care is asymmetrical. When this work takes place in the context of a relationship, however, the asymmetry counts differently.

This ethic of extensive responsibility will encounter objections such as those Joan Tronto has leveled against what she calls "the 'morality first' view" of care.[21] Tronto criticizes advocates of care such as Nell Noddings who assert the primacy of moral values over the political realities of "gaining power and preserving it through force and strength." She characterizes "morality first" positions as maintaining that only "after moral views are fixed, [should] right-thinking individuals suggest to the state how political life should conform to these moral principles" (7).

Tronto advocates the centrality of care to social life, but she also forces the question of whether a morality of care can ever have any practical currency outside of particular communities that define themselves in "morality first" terms. Her question is appropriate to arguments such as those of Mairs and Hilfiker, which rest on an explicitly spiritual faith. Tronto asks whether such an ideal of care can be "sufficiently broad [as a] moral idea to solve the problems of distance, inequality, and privilege" (158).

Some witness to the practical reality of a "morality first" ideal of care is found in Timothy Diamond's report of working as a nursing assistant in Chicago nursing homes. Here, certainly, is the worst paid, most demanding, most asymmetrical, and physically hardest work of care. Yet Diamond discovers real relations of caring. He quotes one of the assistants he works alongside; she explains to him how she performs the literal "dirty work" she does: "'After a while when you get to know these folks, it's like your baby,' she said with a smile. 'You'll find out whose shit stinks and whose don't.'" Diamond calls this remark "framed in a narrative of relationships." These relationships, he writes, "were not something distinct from the work but integral to how it got accomplished."[22]

How does this "narrative of relationships" come about? One interpretation is that the communicative body can be heard *even* in the conditions Diamond describes. The alternative is that these conditions—as opposed to higher status intensive care units—are *exactly where* we should expect to hear the communicative body. On either account, idealism about care is justified. Nursing assistants exemplify Bauman's postmodern moral person. Higher qualified nurses only administer the homes: their orientation is to "the Idea" of keeping charts and state-required accounts of care, such as records of meals and baths (120). The orientation of the nursing assistants is to the well-being and dignity of their patients.

When Diamond asks a fellow worker why she does not get a higher paying job, "her back arched and her eyes blazed. 'This is what I *do*,' she said indignantly, with a quick glance at the person whose face she was washing" (46). She might also have said that this is who she *is*: someone who dedicates her body to helping other bodies.

The example of Diamond's nursing assistants does not obviate Tronto's reservations about "morality first" arguments. Nothing the nursing assistants do will *change* the conditions of their work, and their work can only palliate, not change, the degraded lives of the residents of these nursing homes. The oppressive conditions Diamond describes will persist despite the relations of care that take place within them. Ultimately, moral values require a complementary politics with attention to inequalities of power. But improvement in nursing homes— real change for both nursing assistants and residents—can only come when moral views are changed. Diamond's ethnography shows how nursing homes reflect a society with a primary value of warehousing unwanted "others" at minimal cost. He demonstrates that bureaucratic changes—such as increased state surveillance of living conditions—do not improve the lives of residents and those who care for them. Political change without moral reorientation only adds bureaucracy.

Change will only come when people—families, taxpayers, and voters—care about conditions in nursing homes; when residents and nursing assistants are afforded the fullest respect as persons. The pedagogy of suffering *is* a "morality first" argument, aimed at achieving that shift in moral orientation and thus in political priority.

What is at issue in an ethic derived from a pedagogy of suffering was stated in 1909 by György Lukács, as he meditated on the mysterious reciprocity between creative activity and "the primacy of ethics in life":

> Perhaps the greatest life-value of ethics is precisely
> that it is a sphere where a certain kind of communion
> can exist, a sphere where the eternal loneliness stops.
> The ethical man is no longer the beginning and the
> end of all things, his moods are no longer the
> measure of the significance of everything that
> happens in the world. Ethics forces a sense of
> community upon all men.[23]

The impetus of ethics for Lukács is loneliness; Gail, with her chronic pain that cannot be diagnosed or treated, knows loneliness; so does Mairs, facing both widowhood and complete disability. The nursing assistants confront the loneliness of the residents they care for, and in many cases know loneliness in their own lives as immigrants, and as women of color, who are economically disadvantaged and occupationally marginal. The pedagogy of suffering begins its teaching from a ground of loneliness seeking communion. This communion is the reward of the nursing assistant who cleans the soiled resident and claims it does not stink because of the relationship between them.

The promise of the ethics Lukács recommends is that it lightens the load on people. The ethical person he imagines is "no longer the beginning and end of all things." Being the beginning and end of all things—having to settle the hash of the universe—is the weight modernity puts on its heroes. Physicians feel this weight. Because hospitals and medical offices are run on the assumption that the doctor's mood is "the measure of significance of everything that happens in the world," the doctor has to bear that weight. The danger of imagining ill people as heroes is putting this same weight on them; the Phoenix as an expectation becomes a burden, not a liberation.

The community Lukács recommends spreads the weight around. Once the moral person has acknowledged his own lack, service is necessary but also easier. All that is needed is to serve the other person. "Not all of us who work with the poor are saints," writes David Hilfiker, "but maybe we don't have to be. Perhaps sainthood isn't a prerequisite for the job."[24] This easing of burdens having been recommended, burdens remain. The problem of replacing liability, especially limited liability, with responsibility is burn out. Hilfiker reports his own eventual burn out (256) and with characteristic honesty notes that his own "safety net" allowed him to go elsewhere and take time off. The nursing assistants lack that option.

The examples of the nursing assistants and of David Hilfiker demonstrate that ill bodies have no special privilege as moral persons; others can become communicative bodies just as well. Illness is *only one form of pedagogy* that can teach the need to become a moral person. What ill people and those who are often the lowest level of their caregivers—whether nursing assistants or practitioners of poverty medicine—have in common is a kind of desperate necessity.

The communicative body is a choice that derives from necessity, and the pedagogy of suffering describes this necessity. When an illusion of oneself as the beginning and end of all things can no longer be maintained, then openness to communion is all that is left. Many faith communities believe in the curious alchemy that whoever engages in that communion thus becomes the beginning and end of all things.

NARRATIVE ETHICS

Because the pedagogy of suffering is taught in the testimony of illness stories, the kind of ethic it supports is a narrative ethic.

The question such an ethic poses is the core of what this book is about: how are lives to be affected by stories?

Narrative ethics is a term with some currency in the field of ethics and health care. Describing this work, Rita Charon argues convincingly that "narrative ethics is not an independent method that promises to replace all existing efforts in the field of medical ethics."[25] What Charon calls medical ethics began as "a project of administering universally applicable principles and adjudicatory rules to health care conflicts" (260). She points out that ethics currently goes well beyond this scope and "increasingly has come to include the search for the meanings of singular human situations" (260), but her concern remains with "the practice of the ethicist" (her subtitle) in resolving "health care conflicts."

Charon suggests how the study of narrative—what I would call narrative sensitization—can contribute to improving the "trustworthiness of medical ethics." Such study would help caregivers:

first, "to recognize the narrative coherence, however obscured, of the patient's life";

second, to identify "multiple tellers of the patient's story, the several audiences to whom the story is told, and the interpretive community responsible for understanding it";

third, "to examine contradictions among the story's multiple representations, conflicts among tellers and listeners, and ambiguities in the events themselves";

and fourth, to help all participants in ethical deliberations to appreciate "the coherence, the resonance, and the singular meaning of particular human events" (261).[26]

Charon is a physician, and her concern—properly for a physician—is with "the patient." For her, the value of "narrative contributions" lies in their ability to enhance medical caregivers' recognition of the complexity of treatment decisions. As such, narrative plays a crucial but ancillary role: by leading physicians to recognize the moral dimension in *every* medical encounter (264), it helps to ground difficult medical decisions in the concreteness and specificity of each patient's life.

Certainly, the reading of published illness stories can lead to the "narrative contributions" to medical decision-making that Charon imagines. It is, however, in the realm *beyond* clinical medical encounters that narrative ethics becomes a distinct activity. In the chapters above I have interpreted illness stories with the goal of enhancing the hearing of stories that might not otherwise be heard, or might be treated as "just" conversational with no clinical or ethical import. These stories open up moral dimensions of the lives of ill persons when they are *not* being patients.

If a unique sphere can be claimed for narrative ethics, this sphere is illness outside patienthood. Clinical ethics is concerned primarily with professional and institutional obligations to patients. But with the increasing proportions of chronic and degenerative diseases, more ill people spend more of their time not being patients; what I call "the remission society" grows. The ethical questions for members of the remission society are not adjudications of health care conflicts but *how to live a good life while being ill.* The cornerstones of this "good life" involve those same decisions that I identified with respect to living in a body, especially desire. The core ethical questions concern what the ill person should want for herself and for others. As ethical questions, desires become responsibilities: what is it *good* to want for oneself and others?

Medical and other professional caregivers are hardly excluded from this narrative ethics, but neither are they involved in their core professional capacities. As professionals, their concern is closer to what Charon describes: helping *patients* live good lives with the aid of appropriate treatments. Medical work, however, has another side, when the professional-patient relationship becomes a relationship of two persons.

Arthur Kleinman describes being asked by a patient who had suffered multiple losses and was seriously ill, "Can you give me the courage I need?"[27] The question is not a request for medical information or treatment; Kleinman hears himself being called to a moral relationship in Levinas's sense of being *for*-another. However he responds to this question, his medical expertise is minimally relevant. The woman is asking Kleinman if he, as a person, can be *for* her, as a person. The ethic of his response involves not a health care conflict—the paradigm occasion for clinical ethics—but the assumption of a profound moral commitment.[28] Narrative ethics guides people, whether ill or healthy, lay or professional, in the moral commitments that illness calls them to.

Thus I am less concerned with the significant narrative contributions to ethics that Charon describes so well. Nor am I concerned with narrative ethics as ethicists' practice of "thick description" of cases.[29] My concern is with ill people's self-stories as moral acts, and with care as the moral action of responding to those self-stories. The *ethics* in narrative ethics is best suggested by Barry Hoffmaster: "The crucial test of a story might be the sort of person it shapes."[30]

Hoffmaster intends this test as a limitation on narrative ethics which he, like Charon, views as incomplete by itself. His valid argument is that this test "presupposes that one already knows the difference between good and bad, or virtuous and non-virtuous persons" (1161). My response, perhaps more postmodern, is that because one *never* knows these differences in advance or even in retrospect,[31] narrative ethics has no inherent limitation that is not shared in any other ethical inquiry. The advantage of narrative is to confront this uncertainty head on. Narrative teaches that being human is the perpetual finding out of what is good and virtuous, whether the process of that moral inquiry is called the examined life or reflexive monitoring.

The moral imperative of narrative ethics is perpetual self-reflection on the sort of person that one's story is shaping one into, entailing the requirement to change that self-story if the wrong self is being shaped. Thus awareness of the general type of narrative one is telling or responding to—restitution, chaos, or quest—is a crucial beginning.

Narrative ethics is complete, within its sphere. This sphere is not clinical adjudication but personal becoming. Narrative ethics is an ethics of commitment to shaping oneself as a human being. Specific stories are the media of this shaping, and the shaping itself is the story of a life.

¤   ¤   ¤

Thinking *with* stories is the basis of narrative ethics. The physician may take her patient's story seriously, but only to hear a truth that the patient himself cannot tell. The corrected story becomes the "case." Cases are objects of professional scrutiny. In presentations of cases, professionals talk *about* people's stories; the story is an object of analysis, and professionals believe themselves to be the only ones qualified to carry out this analysis.[32] If Kleinman had heard his patient's question, "Can you give me the courage I need?" exclusively as a professional, his response would have been to wonder about possible medication for a diagnosable depression. He would have missed the opening to a relationship.

Thinking with stories means joining with them; allowing one's own thoughts to adopt the story's immanent logic of causality, its temporality, and its narrative tensions. Narrative ethics seeks to remain with the story, even when it can no longer remain inside the story. The goal is empathy, not as internalizing the feelings of the other, but as what Halpern calls "resonance" with the other.[33] The other's self-story does not become my own, but I develop sufficient resonance with that story so that I can feel its nuances and anticipate changes in plot.

reflexive monitoring

But the primary question is not how to think with the other's story; it is how to think with your *own* story. Or, how is narrative ethics a practice of reflexive monitoring for the ill themselves?

As I hear Native Canadians speak of their stories and what it means to live in an oral culture, I am struck by their *retelling* of stories. When stories are retold, the point is not what is learned from their content, any more than the point of Gail's experience can be stated in so many analytical points. The point is rather what a listener *becomes* in the course of listening to the story. Repetition is the medium of becoming. Professional culture has little space for personal becoming. Young doctors are not trained to think of the careers ahead of them as trajectories of their own moral development, which is one reason why they have trouble with an expanded notion of service.

Professionals understand stories as something to carry a message away *from*—as in, "What did you learn from that history?" The professional, as paradigmatic modernist, is always moving on, the sooner to get to the next thing and move on from that. The danger for ill people is that they are often taught how to be ill by professionals. Illness is not presented to the ill as a moral problem; people are not asked, after the shock of diagnosis has dulled sufficiently, what do you wish to *become* in this experience? What story do you wish to tell of yourself? How will you shape your illness, and yourself, in the stories you tell of it?

The first lesson of thinking with stories is not to move on once the story has been heard, but to continue to live in the story, *becoming* in it, reflecting on who one is becoming, and gradually modifying the story. The problem is truly to *listen* to one's own story, just as the problem is truly to listen to others' stories.

Thinking with stories also requires attending to how a story is *used* on different occasions of its telling. As the same story is repeated on different occasions over years and decades, people hear it differently. In its repetition, the story provides continuity between different occasions of the body-self's life.

At some point, however, continuity gives way to unfathomable difference. "In the end, he imagines that he might live a different story and that words have taken him only to the 'threshold of my story, before the door that opens on my story,'" writes Martha Nussbaum, quoting Samuel Beckett's *The Unnameable.*[34] What the story teaches is that there is always another story, and other stories have always been possible. One meaning of this lesson is that life is lived in decisions, each setting in place a different way of telling the story. Because these decisions have consequences—the plot cannot be reversed at will at any point—they are moral.

Thinking with stories means that narrative ethics cannot offer people clear guidelines or principles for making decisions. Instead, what is offered is permission to *allow the story to lead in certain directions.* Medical workers need this permission. When physicians in an intensive care unit present a case to me, I can only ask questions about who their patients are, how the present illness fits into the pattern of these people's lives, and where both the physicians and the patients' families see their pattern leading. In intensive care situations the ill person is often mute, as an effect of disease, medication, or life-support mechanisms. But despite being unable to speak to the patient, the medical staff usually have a good idea of the story. I offer them permission to invoke this narrative knowledge to make professional decisions.

Some of the most unfortunate medical decisions are made when there is a breakdown in the continuity of relationship and of story. In his early exploration of narrative ethics, Steven Miles wrote of an elderly nursing home resident whose imminent death precipitated transfer to a hospital where no one knew her. The nursing home staff who did know her wishes were no longer making the decisions, and life-support measures were instituted that the woman would not have wanted. Physicians who knew nothing of her life could not try to achieve the kind of death that made sense as the culmination of that life.[35]

But ill people do not tell their stories so that medical workers can make decisions. Self-stories are told to make sense of a life that has reached some moral juncture. Nearing the end of his "sort of memoir," Stewart Alsop writes that he is about to turn sixty; after an interval of almost thirty pages he adds that "perhaps this is a good time to bow out."[36] In order to think with Alsop's story, and perhaps to be guided by that story in some future decision, narrative ethics might pose this question: What is said in between these statements to connect them, and what narrative work does Alsop have to do to make the latter follow as a *sequitur* to the former? Other people might consider life to be beginning a new stage at sixty and thus interpret illness differently.

In between observing turning sixty and accepting bowing out, Alsop tells a series of anecdotes from his experiences as a young officer in World War II. He marries an even younger English woman, who is happily still his wife as he writes. They enjoy a honeymoon that was as lavish as London during the bombing could provide; its memory becomes more mythic because of that bombing. Alsop leaves his bride to participate in a failed parachute landing in occupied France, and by a series of remarkably lucky coincidences he escapes being captured. These stories connect turning sixty with bowing out, and they establish a direction for ethical decision-making, by rendering the incoherence of Alsop's disease and imminent death coherent.

Alsop was not supposed to end up dying at sixty; leukemia is a tragic and frustrating imposition on his life. His wartime anecdotes address the incoherence of cancer in at least this way: if Alsop is to die at sixty, he has had an extraordinary sixty years.

He might well have died in the London bombing or in the parachute raid. If he lived through these by a series of accidents, there is no particular injustice to his dying now because of some equally accidental events in his bloodstream. The continuity of Alsop's self is reestablished as the story of someone who has always lived by his luck. If the event of his illness remains tragic, it nevertheless takes on an acceptable level of rightness.

The wartime stories reinforce this rightness in another way as well. These stories have probably been told and retold in the Alsop family. The stories are the core mythology of Alsop's marriage, its touchstone. I imagine them having been used on different occasions for different purposes: sometimes as diversions and entertainments, other times to remind Alsop and his wife who they were together and what they had come through, yet other times to teach children who their family is.

Now Alsop is telling the old stories on what may be his last occasion. The simple fact that they can be told again, that they still fit the present circumstances, places those circumstances within the continuity of the family's lives together and gives illness a sad but acceptable rightness. Dying is *not* a loss of the old map and destination; in the context of the familiar stories, dying is accepting where the map always led.

Alsop follows his remark about bowing out with the last of many anecdotes concerning Winston Churchill that he tells throughout the book. He describes the old Churchill attending parliament for the last time. To the embarrassed hush of his younger colleagues, he slumps over his desk, dozing. Alsop paints a pathetic picture of the hero as relic, adding the fine epitaph that he has already applied to several others: "He should have died herebefore."[37] Churchill as metaphor becomes the storyline that Alsop rejects for himself; better to bow out than to doze off.

Stewart Alsop is not a "case" to be described as "acceptance" or "denial" or any other reduction of his capacity for moral choice about who he is and how he wants to live. His story, which is really a complex of stories interrupting each other, shows the paucity of such labels. For purposes of ethics, what counts most is that Alsop tells a self-story that gives his dying a sense of rightness for himself and, I hope, for his family as well.

Telling his story is the final discharge of his responsibility. For a caregiver who would enter into a relationship with Alsop, the story invites *becoming the sort of person* who could act within the story in ways that Alsop would appreciate. In terms of the question asked Kleinman, Alsop tells himself how to find the courage he needs, and he shows others where to find the strength to care for him. His story provides for Diamond's "narrative of relationships" between himself and his family and caregivers.

Narrative ethics takes place in telling and listening. There is no such thing as a self-story if that term is taken literally; only self-other-stories. The stories we call "ours" are already bits and pieces we have gathered from others' stories, and we exist no less in their "self"-stories. Ultimately narrative ethics is about recognizing how much we as fellow-humans have to do with each other. As we grope toward some unknowable vision of the good and virtuous, cutting and pasting stories, borrowing and lending along the way, we become communicative bodies.

RECURSION AND RISK

The communicative body, as I wrote when introducing it, is not only an ideal type but an *idealized* one; the ideal of the communicative body grounds criteria for ethical action. Becoming a communicative body is an ethical end, a telos, for a life to aspire to. Because this telos is never fully achieved short of being a Bodhisattva or a Christ, the communicative body is not a fixed state but a *recursive process*. Recursion is what is involved in "pulling yourself up by your own bootstraps"; gravity-defying as that image is, such processes happen.

The communicative body creates itself, recursively, as an ideal that guides choosing which actions can bring itself into being. The simplest analogy is faith: one must have faith in order to be faithful, and being faithful increases the quality of faith. Like faith, the communicative body is always an incomplete project; recursive processes continuously loop, never conclude. I refer to the communicative body using the modernist term "project." Modernist projects imagine their endings before they are begun; their object is completion because modernism seeks to move on to another project as quickly as possible. Postmodernity prefers discovering the nature of the project during the activity of carrying it out.[38] Thus what the communicative body tries to do is to become a communicative body.

The nature of the project changes in postmodern times, but people should not give up on projects.[39] When people lose "The Project" that Frederick Franck calls becoming more fully human, then postmodernity is a moral void. Franck asks, "Could the Meaning of being born human be, to become Human?"[40] This question is too practical to be called rhetorical, but it is too vast to provide for an answer. As a project, it is recursive. Like a story, it can only be lived. What Franck calls becoming Human, I call the communicative body.

The illness story begins in wreckage, having lost its map and destination. The story is both interrupted and it is about interruption. In the illness stories what begins as the breakdown of narrative—life's interruption by illness—is transformed into *another kind* of narrative. I recall one of my great aunts commenting on a piece of popular music. The band was playing the time signature wrong, she said, but they were playing it so consistently wrong that it became their own time signature. A life with serious illness is out of time, if time is measured by the metronome of social expectation. The illness story creates its own time out of interrupted time, or its own coherence out of incoherence.

One reason I return to Stewart Alsop and Audre Lorde is the jumpy, interrupted quality of their writing. In Alsop the interruptions appear seamless; the book transforms interruption into culmination. Lorde gives her interruptions a rougher edge; she wants to preserve the grating immediacy of illness. Both, in their respective ways, are *reclaiming* interruption as theirs to tell.

Only the communicative body can reclaim interruption because only it associates with its own contingent vulnerability. The communicative body makes this contingency the condition of its desire, reaching toward others who share this vulnerability. Here again is recursion: the body grounds the story that in its telling allows the body to realize itself. The body "realizes" itself in the dual senses of gaining self-reflection and of making itself real in action. "Making itself real" figures most significantly in the achievement of character.

The body's story requires a character, but who the character is is only created in the telling of the story. The character who is a communicative body must bear witness; witness requires voice as its medium, and voice finds its responsibility in witnessing. What is witnessed is memory, specifically embodied memory, a memory of experience now written into the tissues. St. Paul, whose attitudes toward sexual embodiment are not popular, nevertheless expressed the embodiment of witness passionately. Paul knows he witnesses through his body: "In stripes, in imprisonments, in tumults, in labours, in watchings, in fastings" (2 Corinthians 6:5). Paul's ministry, to bring others into the body of Christ, is effected through rendering his own body available to suffering. This archetypal affinity of witness and bodily suffering cannot be evaded: Paul's unpopular message is that the responsibility of some is to find themselves called to the nexus of this affinity.

The same voice of embodied witness is heard in Nancy Mairs's writing. She tells a story about an editor of one of her earlier books, whose enthusiasm she had to dampen. Explaining why her book's sales potential would be limited, Mairs tells her editor, "The subtext here is that we are all going to die, and that that's all right. It's not a message that will attract readers in droves." But like any authentic witness, she had no choice in what she wrote: "I had to risk a messenger's death then and still must do: We *are* all going to die. And it *is* all right."[41]

The quest story accepts illness as a calling, a vocation. This vocation includes responsibility for testimony, and testimony implies risk: dying a messenger's death, as Mairs calls it. Risking one's body implies an ethic. The value of this ethic, its witness, is to speak outside of the language of survival. Modernity disallows any language other than survival; the modernist hero cannot imagine any other way to be, which is why physicians are often genuinely baffled by criticisms. People in postmodern times need different languages of meta-survival with various messages that death is all right. Clinical ethics needs these messages.

Audre Lorde, who brought a poet's sense of language to the question of witness, wrote that she and other women together "examined the words to fit a world in which we all believed."[42] Later she writes of translating "the silence surrounding breast cancer into language and action" (61). To make the world she believes in a reality, Lorde must find the words to fit that world.

Lorde expresses most directly the quality of moral humanity that is realized by all those who tell illness stories. At the beginning of her book she writes of her "terror" that if she opens herself to memories of illness, she "might also open myself again to disease." This risk informs her decision to write. Here is the voice of the communicative body, turning interruption into witness: "I had to remind myself that I had lived through it, already. I had known the pain, and survived it. It only remained for me to give it voice, to share it for use, that the pain not be wasted" (16).

This witness is uniquely that of Audre Lorde, but Audre Lorde could only be who she is in postmodern times, and these times are formed by people like Audre Lorde. Her narrative becomes the ethic of her times.

Eight

The Wound as Half Opening

SUFFERING AND RESISTANCE

The unspecified topic of this book has been suffering. My early chapters told how the body's suffering during illness creates a need for stories. The middle chapters described narrative structures in which these sufferings become stories. Stories were then understood as a form of testimony: testimony is initiated by suffering, and suffering comes to understand itself by hearing its own testimony. Finally, an ethical practice based on narrative was proposed.

At the center of narrative ethics is the wounded storyteller. What is ethical is found in the story, and the story depends on the wound. Thus my meta-story returns to the wound itself, to suffering.

The most complete definitions of suffering to be offered recently for clinical purposes are by Eric Cassell and Arthur Kleinman. Cassell makes three points with respect to suffering. First, suffering involves whole persons and thus "requires a rejection of the historical dualism of mind and body." The subject who suffers is, in Kleinman's phrase, a body-self.

Second, suffering takes place when a "state of severe distress . . . threaten[s] the intactness of person." This distress can be immediate or imminent, real or perceived: "Suffering occurs," Cassell writes, "when an impending destruction of the person is perceived; it continues until the threat of disintegration has passed or until the integrity of the person can be restored in some other manner."

Third, and still emphasizing the person as a whole of mind and body, Cassell argues that "suffering can occur in relation to any aspect of the person."[1]

To Cassell's three conditions of suffering a fourth and fifth can be added. Resistance is the fourth condition. Kleinman writes that suffering "is the result of processes of resistance (routinized or catastrophic) to the lived flow of experience." To suffer, a person must not only perceive a threat but must resist that threat. The perception of threat is already a weak form of resistance, since the lived flow of experience is disrupted. But Kleinman's emphasis on resistance opens inquiry to more active resistances than Cassell suggests. Telling stories is a form of resistance. In the story, the flow of experience is reflected upon and redirected; resistance through the self-story becomes the remaking of the body-self.

The fifth condition of suffering is its social nature; the prior four all depict suffering as personal, taking place within the body-self. But Kleinman further argues that suffering is "both an existential universal of human conditions *and* a form of practical and, therefore, novel experience that undergoes great cultural elaboration in distinctive local worlds."[2] As I wrote in the first chapter of this book, people tell uniquely personal stories, but they neither make up these stories by themselves, nor do they tell them only to themselves. Bodies and selves are, in Kleinman's phrase, culturally elaborated.

All illness stories share a common root in suffering as "an existential universal of human conditions"; this commonality of suffering cuts across worlds of race and gender as well as types of disease. Audre Lorde's story has metaphoric parallels with Robert Murphy's (see chapter 6, "Quest as Self-Story"), but the storylines that elaborate these parallel metaphors reflect the differences in the two authors' "distinctive local worlds." Similarly, the difference between Lorde's prophetic indignation and Alsop's patrician resignation is hardly accounted for by different personalities, a term that only requires another question. Their stories are the respective products of the worlds each moves through, though these local worlds are also formed anew with each act of interpretation of every story the community recognizes as theirs. Distinctive local worlds elaborate stories, but stories and their interpretation also integrate local worlds.

The story that the local world elaborates may be written or oral. Women organizing themselves in breast cancer activism have found Audre Lorde's book to be a point of mutual recognition. Families recognize what they share as they elaborate oral stories of members' illnesses and deaths. These elaborations become powerful sources of present solidarity as well as models, whether recommended or cautionary, for others' future illnesses. Thus stories are elaborated in local worlds, but stories also elaborate those worlds.

Stories of suffering have two sides. One side, reflecting Cassell's emphases, expresses the threat of disintegration. The chaos narrative is overwhelmed by this threat; disintegration has become the teller's encompassing reality. The other side, reflecting Kleinman's emphasis on resistance, seeks a new integration of body-self. The quest narrative recognizes that the old intactness must be stripped away to prepare for something new. Quest stories reflect a confidence in what is waiting to emerge from suffering.

The resources for creating a new body-self seem uniquely at hand in postmodern times. To be bombarded with stories also means having a variety of stories at one's disposal. Reclaiming has a popular availability. The road of trials can become a journey because the journey motif is available as a self-definition.

Postmodern ill people thus live simultaneously with both

the threat of disintegration and the promise of reintegration. The body-self whose foreground is dominated by threat is unmade, but unmaking can be a generative process; what is unmade stands to be remade.

THE SELF UNMADE:
EMBODIED PARANOIA

Illness has always threatened the intactness of mind and body, but in postmodern times this threat takes the particular form I have called *embodied paranoia*.[3] The clearest epigram for embodied paranoia is the phrase heard often at public symposia on euthanasia: "I don't want to die on a machine." In postmodern times people fear for their bodies not only from natural threats such as storms or disease and from social threats such as crime or war. People are also threatened by institutions ostensibly designed to help them.

Becoming a victim of medicine is a recurring theme in illness stories. The incompetence of individual physicians is sometimes an issue, but more often physicians are understood as fronting a bureaucratic administrative system that colonizes the body by making it into its "case." People feel victimized when decisions about them are made by strangers.[4] The sick role is no longer understood as a release from normal obligations; instead it becomes a vulnerability to extended institutional colonization.

I use the term embodied *paranoia* to suggest the internal conflicts that attend this fear of colonization; what is involved is more complex than simple fear for one's body. Even war and crime are "natural" threats in the sense that they are intended to harm and fear of them is natural. Fearing institutions that are designed to help is not natural. This fear is *reflectively* paranoid in its self-doubt about whether it ought to be afraid or has a right to be afraid. The inner conflicts of this reflective paranoia are evident in the troubling analogy between torture and medical treatment.

Some of my deepest, even haunted, discussions with other members of the remission society have been attempts to sort out whether chemotherapy is a form of torture. We know that in most "objective" respects the two situations differ, and we seek only to make sense of our own memories and fears, not to appropriate the far greater suffering of torture victims. But chemotherapy fits with disturbing ease into Elaine Scarry's definition of torture as "unmaking the world."[5] The realization that obsessed me during chemotherapy was how easily every strength I thought I had could be reduced to weakness. I was unmade as my mind sought to hold onto the promise that this treatment was curing me, while my body deteriorated: my intactness, my integrity as a body-self, disintegrated.

"I never thought of myself as ill with cancer," says Marcia in her story. "I was never sick before or after the mastectomy. . . . Not true of chemo; chemo was hell. Chemo was not therapeutic; it produced illness. I hated it. I cried every time I had it and did not trust it at all. I felt so vulnerable."[6] The voice heard here is someone undergoing a kind of torture. In chemotherapy, Marcia's body becomes what Scarry calls "the agent of [her] agony."[7] Her body is, in the treatment, "made to be the enemy" (48). Physicians believe chemotherapy will cure Marcia; she does not. As Scarry writes of torture, "the body belongs to a person other than the person whose body is used to confirm [the belief]" (149). Yet people in chemotherapy also believe that they are being *cared* for. Or they believe they ought to believe this, or they have given up believing but still confront others who insist that their treatment is care. The self is unmade in the opposition of the mind's message of care and the body's message of pain.

Chemotherapy is hardly the only occasion for comparing medical treatment to torture. Intensive care residents observed by Zussman describe their work as torture and feel tortured themselves by what they believe their work requires.[8] Zussman, Klass, and Quill all report the "cheechee" story as standard medical black humor that illustrates physicians' attempts to neutralize the grim realities of their work.[9] The point of the "joke" is to make its telling as grotesque as possible; without those flourishes, the basic plot describes two or more explorers captured by savages. The first explorer is offered a choice of death or cheechee. Not knowing what the latter means, he chooses it and is horribly tortured to death. The second explorer is given the same choice and chooses death. The chief is puzzled at his decision. "All right," he says, "but first, a little cheechee."

Surrendering one's body to the medical world of "limited liability" is frightening: cheechee does happen. The fear of cheechee is complicated, and conflicted, because the high-tech medical world remains the perpetual source of the hope that keeps restitution stories going.[10] Marcia lives to tell her story, although even years later she does not give much credit to chemotherapy. High-tech medicine offers real hopes, and resistance to "dying on a machine" is itself resisted by wanting what that machine might offer. The resistances that Kleinman places at the core of suffering are resistances within and against other resistances.

Embodied paranoia is not knowing what to fear most, and then feeling guilty about this very uncertainty. The patient knows full well that most of those inflicting the torture are sincerely trying to help; thus he cannot hate them, but neither can he offer them the gratitude that the intensity of their efforts seems to demand. Max Lerner reports being mildly reprimanded by his student-physician son for his ambivalent gratitude toward the physicians who administered his chemotherapy. Lerner takes the point but retains his ambivalence: "I

wish however that those who came up with Adriamycin and Cy-
toxan for my advanced large-cell lymphoma might have hit
upon a less bruising mixture," he writes.[11]

The other source of Lerner's ambivalence is that, in chemotherapy, medicine appropriates his healing to itself. Lerner's
healing is *his* story, and he wants it back: "We don't know how
much of the healing was due to the chemical, how much . . . to
the patient who was fighting not only the tumor but, to a de-
gree, the doctors and even the chemotherapies addressed to
the tumors" (57). Lerner's embodied paranoia is not fear of
medicine, yet his reflection on his need to fight his doctors
shows a profound resistance. How he fights is not specified; I
would say Lerner needs to keep the fight his own. Even someone so secure in his own voice senses an appropriation he must
resist. Other post-colonial selves hear the medical narratives
that claim to tell their stories for them as reflecting the interests of corporations, bureaucracies, and hyphenated "-indus-
trial" complexes of different kinds: medical care becomes the
health care industry.

But if the post-colonial self no longer wants itself to be told
in narratives from elsewhere, neither does this self have substitute narratives of its own immediately available. In postmodern
times subjection to colonizing narratives—the oppressive side
of Keen's condition of being bombarded by stories (see chapter
3)—can never be fully escaped.

Disease and treatment happen to a body-self that is already
substantially unmade by a combination of embodied paranoia
and post-colonial skepticism. With respect to Cassell's main
condition of suffering, postmodern times place the embodied
self in a *perpetual* condition of multiply threatened intactness.
Disease is all too effective as a journalistic metaphor for social
problems—crime, poverty, drug use, inflation—because disease metaphors tap the intuitive connection between internal

threats to the body and external threats. Embodied paranoia reflects a blurring of internal and external: everything has potential to threaten.

When illness happens, the disease carries a metonymic overload that compounds suffering. The disease is fully real in itself; the tip of the iceberg is still real ice. *And* the disease is a part standing for a larger whole, the external threats. Some of these threats, like fear of "cheechee," are related to the disease, while other fears of being made a victim have no necessary relation but are summoned up nonetheless. The losses brought by the disease open up extensive fears that one's intactness has always been more imaginary than the self has wanted to believe.

Selves truly are unmade in these complex fears, but the same unmaking processes can elicit different responses. If one cannot control what happens, these events can still be lived in different ways. Paul Ricoeur intimates a sort of resolution when he writes of "becoming the narrator of our own story without becoming the author of our life."[12] In the context of Ricoeur's biblical hermeneutics, his statement seems to refer to faithful acceptance of divine authorship. In postmodern times, becoming a narrator of one's own life implies an assumption of responsibility for more than the events of that life. Events *are* contingent, but a story can be told that binds contingent events together into a life that has a moral necessity.

REMAKING THE BODY-SELF

Remaking begins when suffering becomes an opening to others. Emmanuel Levinas presents perhaps the darkest vision of suffering as what I have called monadic self-enclosure. Because pain "isolates itself in consciousness, or absorbs the rest of consciousness," suffering is, literally, a dead end: "useless, 'for nothing' . . . this basic sense-lessness."[13] Yet these very depths seem the precondition for a new impulse. Levinas describes this remaking:

> Is not the evil of suffering—extreme passivity, impotence, abandonment and solitude—also the unassumable and thus the possibility of a half opening, and, more precisely, the possibility that wherever a moan, a cry, a groan or a sigh happen there is the original call for aid, for curative help, for help from the other ego whose alterity, whose exteriority promises salvation? . . . For pure suffering, which is intrinsically meaningless and condemned to itself without exit, a beyond takes shape in the inter-human. (158)

The orientation that Levinas calls the inter-human becomes possible—or as I suggested in the first chapter, once again becomes news—at a precise historical moment, "the end of a century of nameless suffering" (159). Levinas enumerates "two world wars, the totalitarianisms of right and left, Hitlerism and Stalinism, Hiroshima, the Gulag, and the Genocides of Auschwitz and Cambodia" (162), and since he wrote the list goes on. At this historical moment when consciousness is overwhelmed with "unjustifiable" sufferings, the sense of suffering splits.

On one side is the suffering that Levinas calls, in the above quotation, "unassumable," which I take to mean the suffering that the individual cannot assume as his own; he cannot give his own suffering any meaning, and no other person can assume this suffering for him. This *"suffering in the Other"* can only be witnessed as "unpardonable" (159). This suffering "solicits me and calls me," eliciting in me "a suffering for the suffering." Thus a second order of suffering begins: "a just suffering in me for the unjustifiable suffering of the Other." This just suffering can "take on a meaning." This meaning is "attention to the Other," which Levinas calls "the very bond of human subjectivity, even to the point of being raised to a supreme ethical principle" (159).

Out of this profoundest moral darkness, a new light—even if the new light of an old ethic—begins to shine. Suffering becomes "the possibility of a half opening" to the other. As I read Levinas, this opening does not give meaning to the nameless suffering, but neither does that suffering remain useless. The meaning and the just suffering are experienced by the witness. The original, "unassumable" suffering has use in calling the witness to these ethical feelings, but Levinas seems too realistic to believe that it is mitigated.

Levinas's argument suggests a stronger connection between the chaos narrative and the quest narrative. The chaos narrative is the unassumable, nameless suffering. Chaos suffering is "useless" because the chaos story cannot be told, because it is an anti-narrative, a non-self-story. The quest narrative is the just suffering; what Levinas calls "my own adventure of suffering" (159). But the adventure, or journey, is of course not my own. The journey begins as the hero's own, but what the hero learns throughout the journey is that she suffers for others. The boon is a vision of the inter-human. The hero who has returned embodies this "supreme ethical principle." The Bodhisattva and the Christ both return, and their return is the measure of their love of the world.

Most heroes are called to the quest not by their recognition of the suffering of others, which seems to be what calls Levinas, but by their own suffering. The journey is a process of learning that their own suffering touches and is touched by the suffering of others. The "inter-human" opens when suffering becomes the call and response implicating self and other.

One of my conflicts in writing this book was whether to include types of suffering other than illness, particularly whether to include Holocaust sufferings. To discuss these sufferings beside illness necessarily implies comparability or comparison.

There can be no comparison of levels of pain, of the impotence and abandonment, or of the cries, groans, and sighs that Levinas refers to. Comparisons are impossible either between the ill and the nameless sufferings that Levinas enumerates, or among the ill themselves.

Suffering becomes useless precisely because any person's suffering is irreducible: being nothing more than what it is, suffering can have no meaning. Irreducible sufferings can never be compared. But here the argument turns on itself. Once it is understood that sufferings cannot be compared, then it *is* possible to speak of different sufferings in the same story, because there is no comparison. Beyond comparison, the "existential universal" of suffering requires that different forms be spoken of. Where there can be no comparison, there is metonymic overload. Each suffering is part of a larger whole; each suffering person is called to that whole, as a witness to other sufferings.

I also realize that part of my hesitation to speak of illness and the nameless sufferings in the same text is an aspect of my own embodied paranoia. I have this idea that illness is always cared for, or at least ought to be cared for, and thus it cannot be compared to sufferings that are humanly intended to inflict pain. But body-selves are unmade in all sufferings. If suffering is pain that isolates itself in consciousness, absorbing the rest of consciousness, then the true difference is not between suffering that occurs in a hospital and suffering in a concentration camp. The difference is between suffering that has its cry attended to, and suffering that is left in its own uselessness. Again the argument turns on itself: certainly among sufferings illness is far more often responded to; the cry from the camp is stifled.

Levinas's most important lesson is that for everyone rendered "other" by suffering who speaks, perhaps in that act of witness some nameless suffering is opened. The suffering person is always the other, reduced and isolated. To tell any story of suffering is to claim some relation to the inter-human. Any testimony is a response to the half opening of nameless suffering.

I value Levinas's qualification that the opening is only a "half opening." The quest of finding meaning in suffering can only be undertaken oneself; to prescribe this quest to others is arrogance. Levinas requires us to remember the suffering that remains useless, nameless, and untouched; useless but also, in its call to others, not useless. The tragedy is that such suffering will never hear the response to its call. The chaos story remains monadic in its self-enclosure, even as the quest story—the suffering that has found terms to assume what it suffers—calls out to it.

The call for illness stories is more than what I described it to be in chapter 3. There I wrote of the practical imperative to tell people what was happening, and the existential imperative to find a new map and destination. Levinas requires we hear a third level of call: the opening to the inter-human. The Other who suffers now speaks but cannot hear his own speech, because to be able to hear oneself is already to have found some meaning in useless suffering. But this speech that cannot hear itself remains a call for aid. The voiceless are given a voice.

I also suggested above that the parent for the quest story is Nietzsche, who named his pain and thus gave it a use, making it an opening for himself and to others. I now add a much earlier parent, the biblical patriarch Jacob who wrestled with the angel, was wounded in his hip, and persevered until he received a blessing (Genesis 32:24–30). Jacob's story contains the elements of any illness story that brings suffering out of uselessness.

First, the self is formed through *uses of the body*. Jacob wrestles with all his body, and he is wounded in his body. He leaves the scene with a limp, which is the stigmata of his encounter with the divine, and with a new name, Israel, which is the boon of this encounter. The boon is purchased with the wound; the self is thus found through the body, hence the body-self.

Second, the body-self is also a *spiritual* being. Jacob's story is about the complexity of resistance to what readers of the story can only call God. God is the mystery of what Jacob wrestles with; this mystery is not named until the end of the story. Whether Jacob knew at first who he wrestled with, who his attacker was, is unclear.[14] Jacob's impulse toward what is retrospectively known as God is curiously expressed as resistance: Jacob contests the divine. What is being contested remains ambiguous: is Jacob wrestling a blessing out of the angel, or is the angel wrestling the petition for a blessing out of Jacob? Or is Jacob wrestling in order to be wounded, since that wound will finally open him to the spiritual aspect of life he has resisted ever since he stole the blessing that belonged to his brother?

Third, the wounded, spiritual body-self exists in moments of *immanence.* Humans are not alone, even if being with God is a process of resistance, contest, and wound. In his embodied resistance and through his wound, Jacob discovers that he has been on holy ground. As he leaves he "called the place Peniel," which is translated as "the face of God." The face of God was not self-evident in the place when Jacob went to sleep there, deeply troubled and as often in his life, running away. The holiness of the ground is created in the wrestling that sanctifies the ground.

Later in Levinas's essay on suffering he takes up the question of theodicy: how can a just and powerful God allow such sufferings? He responds: "To renounce after Auschwitz this God absent from Auschwitz . . . would amount to finishing the criminal enterprise of National-Socialism, which aimed at the annihilation of Israel and the forgetting of the ethical message of the Bible, which Judaism bears."[15] Peniel is a place where

Jacob may have thought God was absent; he learns in his wounding that God is present. In Peniel, Jacob is renamed Israel.

Finally, the spiritual body-self assumes an ongoing *responsibility.* Jacob leaves Peniel to *be* Israel. The postmodern Jacob describes sanctification as proceeding recursively: resistance is never worked out once and for all; the self must continue to wrestle and continue to be wounded in order to rediscover the ground it now stands on as sacred. *To be is to wrestle with God.*

The illness story accepts what has happened as an ongoing responsibility. Oliver Sacks's claim to be changed is a commitment to continue a process of change. Audre Lorde is a modern Bodhisattva: she commits herself to continue writing until all who are silent are able to speak. Sacks's and Lorde's quest stories are responses to their own moments of chaos; the quest narrative does not stand apart from the chaos narrative but bears witness to it. Nor is the restitution narrative without its responsibility. The call for aid that emanates from nameless suffering is heard by Levinas as "the original opening toward what is helpful, where the primordial, irreducible, and ethical, anthropological category of the medical comes" (158).[16] Cure is life, and life is the fundamental quest.

For wounded storytellers, the return from illness brings the responsibility to teach others so that not only sick people can "know what health is," as Gail says.[17] Neither Sacks, nor Lorde, nor Gail accept their stories without resistance, but their resistance changes. First they resist the call: the disease, or trauma, or chronic pain that is being forced upon their bodies. As their stories develop and as they develop in their stories, they resist the silence that suffering forces upon their body-selves. Finally their resistance finds a voice; they make suffering useful. In the wounds of their resistances, they gain a power: to tell, and even to heal.

A complementary voice to Levinas is Rachel Naomi Remen,

writing as both a member of the remission society and as a physician. Remen describes the wounded healer: "My wound evokes your healer. Your wound evokes my healer. My wound enables me to find you with your wound where you have the illusion of having become lost."[18] The wound is a source of stories, as it opens both in and out: *in,* in order to hear the story of the other's suffering, and *out,* in order to tell its own story. Listening and telling are phases of healing; the healer and the storyteller are one. The healing may not cure the body, but it does remedy the loss of body-self intactness that Cassell identifies with suffering. The sufferer is made whole in hearing the other's story that is also hers, and in having her own story not just be listened to but heard as if it were the listener's own, which it is. The illusion of being lost is overcome.

This chapter has said too much and told too little. In narrative ethics, if the point of a story is not clear, don't explain, tell another story. If what it means to take a place in a story that has been resisted is still not clear, then a final story can be told. Dennis Kaye worked as a logger and freight hauler on the coast of British Columbia until he developed Amyotrophic Lateral Sclerosis, sometimes known as Lou Gehrig's disease. He has lived years longer than doctors predicted and has used those years to become a leading spokesperson for people with ALS.

Kaye ends the story of his life and illness by describing himself sitting on his deck, almost immobile in his wheelchair, watching the herring school in the bay below. All the creatures of the sea come to feed on the fish: seagulls and terns, eagles, herons, even an Orca cow and two calves.

> Even for someone who has spent most of his life
> around the water, it was an inspiration. At its peak,
> the whole scene changed from one of frenzy, greed,
> and pandemonium to one of harmony and balance. It
> was spring itself—everything in its place—each

creature keeping time to a universal pulse. Even the unseen carnage below the surface seemed to be part of something perfect, and I felt a part of that perfection. The sea was alive. The air was alive. And sappy as it sounds, I felt more alive than I had in years.[19]

The depiction is another metaphor that is actually a story-line. In the story of the herring and the pandemonium of animals feeding on them, Kaye both tells a story, and he discovers his own story.

The carnage in the sea is also taking place in Kaye's body, which he says a couple of paragraphs later is "literally starting to fall apart." But Dennis Kaye's grace is to hear the universal pulse within his own dying. He remains fully alive even to his own destruction because what Buddhists would call his "little mind," his personal ego, dissolves into the "big mind." He is dying sooner than later; he learns that his dying will be part of the same springtime when herring school and are eaten. Like Nancy Mairs, he knows that we will all die, and that is all right.

Kaye is not just sitting on his deck, or perhaps he is able to understand what he sees from his deck because of his other work. He organized a support and advocacy organization, ALS Awareness. In this organization Kaye brought together an interpretive community that could understand each other's stories. His story is the forming of this community, which is local in its shared interpretations if not in its geography. The community then elaborates his story, both within itself and beyond. In this elaboration, the community recognizes what it has in common, and it grows. Witness, here as elsewhere, grows in concentric circles.

Dennis Kaye's story has not become a best-seller; as Mairs could tell him, the subtext is wrong. Like most returning heroes, he finds that others do not want his woundedness; they do not want reminders of their own wounds. But to those who know they are wounded, to members of the remission society, Kaye's story is an opening that heals. In his epiphany of participation in the perfection of the universal pulse, he reenchants his life. To those who listen to his story, he reenchants all life.

The wounded storyteller is a moral witness, reenchanting a disenchanted world. In the voices of these storytellers William James's really real speaks clearly; we are reminded of the duties owed to the commonsense world. Postmodern times may be pandemonium, but they are not a void. Illness stories provide glimpses of the perfection.

Notes

Epigraph

1. Quoted in Lawrence Langer, *Holocaust Testimonies: The Ruins of Memory* (New Haven: Yale University Press, 1991), 89.

Preface

1. Henri Nouwen, *The Wounded Healer* (New York: Image Books, 1990).

2. Arthur Kleinman, *The Illness Narratives: Suffering, Healing, and the Human Condition* (New York: Basic Books, 1988), 211ff.; Larry Dossey, *Beyond Illness: Discovering the Experience of Health* (Boulder: Shambhala, 1984), 193ff.; Bill Moyers, *Healing and the Mind* (New York: Doubleday, 1993), 315ff.

3. Rita Charon, "The Narrative Road to Empathy," in Howard Spiro, Mary G. McCrea Curnen, Enid Peschel, and Deborah St. James, eds., *Empathy and the Practice of Medicine: Beyond Pills and the Scalpel* (New Haven: Yale University Press, 1994), 158.

4. Søren Kierkegaard, *Either/Or, Part II*, ed. and trans. Howard V. Hong and Edna H. Hong (Princeton: Princeton University Press, 1987), 260.

5. Charles Lemert, ed., *Social Theory: The Multicultural and Classic Readings* (Boulder: Westview Press, 1993), 1.

1. When Bodies Need Voices

1. Personal communication. All attributed quotations are used by permission. Unattributed quotations, where the speaker/writer was not available to give permission, may be altered to preclude identification.

2. Here and below I seek to adhere as much as possible to established usage that differentiates the "disease" as a physiological process from the "illness" as a social experience of that disease. Yet my attempt to consider illness stories as embodied also deconstructs the distinction: the illness experience is an experience in and of a diseased body. This book is about the precariousness of the accepted thinking, as well as of the professional and institutional practices, that too strictly separate disease from illness.

3. Martin Buber, *I and Thou*, trans. Ronald Gregor Smith (New York: Scribners, 1958), 6.

4. An excellent popularization of scientific research is found in the interviews with Candace Pert (177–93) and David Felton (213–37) in Bill Moyers, *Healing and the Mind* (cf. Preface, n. 2). The social implications of what can be called mind/body research have been developed furthest in cognitive science, in particular: George Lakoff and Mark Johnson, *Metaphors We Live By* (Chicago: University of Chicago Press, 1980), Mark Johnson, *The Body in the Mind: The Bodily Basis of Meaning, Imagination, and Reason* (Chicago: University of Chicago Press, 1987), George Lakoff, *Women, Fire, and Dangerous Things: What Categories Reveal about the Mind* (Chicago: University of Chicago Press, 1987), and Mark Johnson, *Moral Imagination: Implications of Cognitive Science for Ethics* (Chicago: University of Chicago Press, 1993).

5. Another point of usage: I have tried to use *story* when referring to actual tales people tell and *narrative* when discussing general structures that comprise various particular stories. But since narratives only exist in particular stories, and all stories are narratives, the distinction is hard to sustain.

6. On the distinction of "postmodernity," as a time period, and "postmodernism," as a style, see Mike Featherstone, "In Pursuit of the Postmodern: An Introduction," *Theory, Culture & Society* 5 (1988): 195–215. Below I use the adjective "modernist" to remind readers that I mean the modern period, not simply what is contemporary. My usage, however, is informed less by academic debates than by popular usage: "postmodernism" is the term I read in my daily paper.

7. Albert Borgmann, *Crossing the Postmodern Divide* (Chicago: University of Chicago Press, 1992).

8. Pierre Bourdieu, *Outline of a Theory of Practice* (Cambridge: Cambridge University Press, 1977), 166.

9. See chapter 4, note 5, below.

10. George S. Bascom, "Sketches From a Surgeon's Notebook," in Spiro et al., *Empathy and the Practice of Medicine*, 29 (cf. Preface, n. 3).

11. The complementary change that marks this side of the postmodern divide is that the medical story is increasingly trumped by the administrative story, but that postmodern trend is the topic for a different book than this one.

12. Arthur W. Frank, *At the Will of the Body: Reflections on Illness* (Boston: Houghton Mifflin, 1991), 138ff.

13. Personal communication.

14. Susan Sontag, *Illness as Metaphor* (New York: Vintage, 1978), 3.

15. Dan Gottlieb, "Patients must insist that Doctors see the Face behind the Ailment," *The Philadelphia Inquirer*, July 4, 1994.

16. Elizabeth Tyson, "Heal Thyself," *Living Fit*, Winter 1994, 38.

17. Claudine Herzlich and Janine Pierret, *Illness and Self in Society* (Baltimore: Johns Hopkins University Press, 1987), 23. Stanley Joel Reiser quotes the Victorian physician Thomas Syderham, "Nature, in the production of disease is uniform and consistent; so much so, that for the same disease in different persons the symptoms are for the most part the same; and the self-same phenomena you would observe in the sickness of a Socrates you would observe in the sickness of a simpleton." The unavoidable implication is that all patients, for diagnostic purposes, might as well be simpletons. Reiser's conclusion is more moderated: "Thus the symptoms that combine patients into populations have become more significant to physicians than the symptoms that separate patients as individuals." ("Science, Pedagogy, and the Transformation of Empathy in Medicine," in Spiro et al., *Empathy and the Practice of Medicine,* 123–24.)

18. Gayatri Chakravorty Spivak, *The Post-Colonial Critic: Interviews, Strategies, and Dialogues,* ed. Sarah Harasym (New York: Routledge, 1990), 73.

19. Susan Bell, "Political Gynecology: Gynecological Imperialism and the Politics of Self-Help," in Phil Brown, ed., *Perspectives in Medical Sociology* (Prospect Heights, Ill: Waveland Press, 1992), 576–86.

20. For another story of lay narratives achieving a collective voice in opposition to orthodox medicine, see Martha Balshem, *Cancer in the Community: Class and Medical Authority* (Washington: Smithsonian Institution Press, 1993).

21. Physicians, who certainly have their own stories, express their version of post-colonialism when they object to having their experiences of caring for patients taken away from them. A physician employed by an HMO says, "I don't want to *manage clients,* I want to *care for patients.* I don't want to hide behind bureaucratic regs and physician assistants. I want to do the caring." Quoted by Kleinman, *The Illness Narratives,* 219 (cf. Preface, n. 2).

22. One indicator of the need for storytelling about illness are "grass roots" publications such as *Expressions: Literature and Art by People with Disabilities and Ongoing Health Problems* (Sefra Kobrin Pitzele, editor; P.O. Box 16294, St. Paul, Minn. 55116-0294) and *Common Journeys* (Leslie Keyes, editor; 4136 43rd Avenue South, Minneapolis, Minn. 55406). Storytelling also takes place in numerous journal writing workshops conducted in all illness support centers I have visited or received information from. The truly post-modern form of storytelling among the ill are electronic messages exchanged in media such as the Internet. An increasing number of specialized "nets" exist for illness stories. On Internet stories, see Faith McLellan, "From Book to Byte: Narratives of Physical Illness," *Medical Humanities Review* 8 (Fall 1994): 9–21.

23. Anthony Giddens, *Self and Society in the Late Modern Age* (Cambridge: Polity Press, 1991), 75.

24. Rainer Maria Rilke, "Archaic Torso of Apollo," *New Poems [1908], The*

Other Part, trans. Edward Snow (San Francisco: North Point Press, 1987), 2. "Du mußt dein Leben ändern."

25. Zygmunt Bauman, *Mortality, Immortality, and Other Life Strategies* (Stanford: Stanford University Press, 1992), 167.

26. Ibid., 42.

27. Michel Foucault, *The History of Sexuality,* vol. 1: *An Introduction* (New York: Vintage, 1978).

28. The classic statement of this lay/professional split remains Eliot Freidson, *Profession of Medicine: A Study of the Sociology of Applied Knowledge* (Chicago: University of Chicago Press, 1970). The fault lines Freidson identified between lay and professional construction of illness have probably become more evident to all, but now need to be complemented by conflicts within each side. Lay people experience conflict between their need for medicine and their mistrust of it; professionals experience a conflict between their desire to participate in their patients' lives and the increasing corporatism and scientism of medicine; see, as examples, the physician quoted above, note 21, as well as many of the statements by physicians in Spiro, *Empathy and the Practice of Medicine.*

29. William James, *Writings: 1902–1910* (New York: Library of America, 1987), 1344.

30. Alan Wolfe, *The Human Difference: Animals, Computers, and the Necessity of Social Science* (Berkeley: University of California Press, 1993), 114.

31. Susan DiGiacomo writes, in the idiom of anthropology but with more general implication, "'Ethnographic practice' must come to mean not only how we do fieldwork and construct ethnographic texts, but how we live our lives" ("Metaphor as Illness: Postmodern Dilemmas in the Presentation of Body, Mind and Disorder," *Medical Anthropology* 14 [1992]: 132).

32. Arthur W. Frank, "For a Sociology of the Body: An Analytical Review," in Mike Featherstone, Mike Hepworth, and Bryan S. Turner, eds., *The Body: Social Process and Cultural Theory* (London: Sage: 1991), 90–96.

33. I have been less attracted to fiction and poetry than to nonfiction prose. Fictional stories of illness are the topic of the journal *Literature and Medicine;* see also Howard Brody, *Stories of Sickness* (New Haven: Yale University Press, 1987).

34. I provide details in my article, "Reclaiming an Orphan Genre: The First-Person Narrative of Illness," *Literature and Medicine* 13, no. 1 (Spring 1994): 18, n. 8. For a study devoted exclusively to published first-person accounts, which she calls "pathographies," including extensive bibliography, see Anne Hunsaker Hawkins, *Reconstructing Illness: Studies in Pathography* (West Lafayette, Ind.: Purdue University Press, 1993). I am unwilling to adopt Hawkins's preferred term for illness stories, "pathographies," because no ill person has ever called her story a "pathography." Medical language differentiates itself by attaching Greek prefixes of "patho." To call people's

stories "pathographies" places them under the authority of the medical gaze: medical interest in these stories is legitimated, and medical interpretations are privileged. Medicine certainly should be attentive to ill people's stories—and few have done more than Hawkins to generate that attention— but physicians must be attentive on ill people's own terms. For additional objections to "pathography," see "Reclaiming an Orphan Genre," note 3. My review of Hawkins is found in *Literature and Medicine* 12 (Fall 1993): 248–52.

35. The complementary problem with oral stories collected as primary data is that ethical considerations usually lead to changing significant details. For this reason among others, Dena S. Davis argues for using published rather than "collected" stories. ("Rich Cases: The Ethics of Thick Description," *Hastings Center Report* 21 [July–August 1991]: 12–17.)

36. The journal's editorial offices are at The Park Ridge Center, 211 East Ontario, Suite 800, Chicago, IL 60611-3215. As of September 1995, *Second Opinion* will be published in a new format as *Making the Rounds in Health, Faith, and Ethics*.

37. Julia Cruickshank, participating in the panel "Learning from Our Elders' Stories: Indigenous Women and the Narrative Tradition." University of Calgary, March 17, 1994.

38. For details of this reading, see "The Pedagogy of Suffering: Moral Dimensions of Psychological Therapy and Research with the Ill," *Theory and Psychology* 2, no. 4 (1992): 467–85.

2. THE BODY'S PROBLEMS
WITH ILLNESS

1. Arthur Kleinman and Joan Kleinman, "How Bodies Remember: Social Memory and Bodily Experience of Criticism, Resistance, and Delegitimation Following China's Cultural Revolution," *New Literary History* 25 (1994): 710–11.

2. Arthur W. Frank, "For a Sociology of the Body: An Analytical Review" (cf. chap. 1, n. 32). See discussions in Chris Shilling, *The Body and Social Theory* (London: Sage, 1993), 93–98, and in Anthony Synnott, *The Body Social: Symbolism, Self and Society* (New York: Routledge, 1993), 239–41.

3. Alfred Schutz refers to ideal types as puppets in *Collected Papers*, vol. 2: *Studies in Social Theory*, ed. Arvid Brodersen (The Hague: Martinus Nijhoff, 1971), 17–18..

4. Erving Goffman, *Stigma: Notes on the Management of Spoiled Identity* (Englewood Cliffs, N.J.: Prentice Hall, 1963).

5. This "affirmation" may, however, be anything but affirmative. Thus a recent "thinly fictionalized, autobiographical novel" describes the author's ileostomy in terms that self-consciously underscore what Goffman calls

spoiled identity: "A plastic bag full of warm shit hang[s] by my side. I hated the bag, even though it had saved my life. I feared what its odour could reveal about me." Quoted in Richard Perry's review of Donna McFarlane's *Division of Surgery*, "Dark-horse Fiction Nominee Offers Fierce Testimony," *The Globe and Mail*, Toronto, November 12, 1994. McFarlane's prose preempts "the bag," regaining control by revealing more than the bag could.

6. In earlier writing I called this problem "self-relatedness." "Self-relatedness" juxtaposes more neatly to the next problem of "other-relatedness," but what I am discussing under this topic is relation to one's self as a body, hence body-relatedness.

7. For a useful review of the positions taken on this question by classical and early Christian writers, see Synnott, *The Body Social*.

8. Bauman, *Mortality, Immortality*, 36 (cf. chap. 1, n. 25).

9. Robert Zussman, *Intensive Care: Medical Ethics and the Medical Profession* (Chicago: University of Chicago Press, 1992), 33.

10. For survey data on alternative medicine usage, see David M. Eisenberg et al., "Unconventional Medicine in the United States," *The New England Journal of Medicine* 328 (January 28, 1993): 246–52. For ethnographic insights, see Fred M. Frohock, *Healing Powers: Alternative Medicine, Spiritual Communities, and the State* (Chicago: University of Chicago Press, 1992). For stories of using alternative healing, see Gilda Radner, *It's Always Something* (New York: Avon Books, 1989) and David A. Tate, *Health, Hope and Healing* (New York: M. Evans and Company, 1989).

11. Originally written in Schweitzer's *On the Edge of the Primeval Forest*. Quoted by Schweitzer in *Out of My Life and Thought: An Autobiography*, trans. Antje Bultmann Lemke (1933; New York: Henry Holt, 1990), 195.

12. Buber, *I and Thou*, 8 (cf. chap. 1, n. 3).

13. For a sociological perspective on the disease model, see Elliot G. Mishler, "Viewpoint: Critical Perspectives on the Biomedical Model," in Elliot G. Mishler et al., eds., *Social Contexts of Health, Illness, and Patient Care* (Cambridge: Cambridge University Press, 1981), 1–23. Larry Dossey, M.D., has been most provocative in his criticisms of medicine's inability to think beyond the monadic body; see his *Meaning and Medicine* (New York: Bantam, 1991) and *Healing Words: The Power of Prayer and the Practice of Medicine* (New York: HarperCollins, 1993). For the conclusions he suggests about how much bodies have to do with each other, Dossey would be regarded as a "fringe" figure by many.

14. Cf. chap. 1, pp. 14–15.

15. Jacques Lacan, *Écrits: A Selection*, trans. Alan Sheridan (New York: Norton, 1977) and *The Four Fundamental Concepts of Psychoanalysis*, ed. Jacques-Alain Miller, trans. Alan Sheridan (New York: Norton, 1978).

16. Dan Wakefield, *Returning: A Spiritual Journey* (New York: Penguin, 1984), 20.

17. Robert Coles, *The Call of Stories: Teaching and the Moral Imagination* (Boston: Houghton Mifflin, 1989), 142.

18. Stewart Alsop, *Stay of Execution: A Sort of Memoir* (Philadelphia: Lippincott, 1973), 288.

19. Malcolm Diamond, "Coping With Cancer: A Funny Thing Happened on My Way to Retirement," *The Princeton Alumni Weekly,* April 6, 1994, 13–16.

20. Anatole Broyard, *Intoxicated by My Illness: And Other Writings on Life and Death,* comp. and ed. Alexandra Broyard (New York: Clarkson N. Potter, 1992), 23.

21. For contemporary statements of the centrality of service to medicine, see Robert Coles, *The Call of Stories,* and David Hilfiker, *Not All of Us Are Saints: A Doctor's Journey with the Poor* (New York: Hill and Wang, 1994).

22. Robert Merton, "Social Structure and Anomie," *American Sociological Review* 3 (October 1938): 672–82.

23. Deborah H. Kahane, *No Less A Woman* (New York: Simon & Schuster, 1990), 118.

24. "Jaco & Jackie O." *Star,* April 5, 1994, 7.

25. The real trauma of hair loss should not be minimized either. Henri Nouwen describes the nearly bald head of the younger son in Rembrandt's painting, "The Return of the Prodigal Son": "When a man's hair is shaved off, whether in prison or in the army, in a hazing ritual or in a concentration camp, he is robbed of one of the marks of his individuality" (*The Return of the Prodigal Son: A Story of Homecoming* [New York: Image Books, 1994], 46). Nouwen does not include hospitals in his list of sites where hair is cut off, but the places he does mention contextualize the experience of hair loss in chemotherapy. And if he refers to a man's loss, how much greater women's loss of individuality must be.

26. Carole E. Andersen, "The Case: Another Side of Cancer," *Second Opinion* 19 (April 1994): 27–31. The original title of Andersen's story was "Some Get Mad," which I suggested based on a phrase she used in an early draft. The editorial shift from "Some Get Mad" to "Another Side of Cancer" exemplifies the way editing can change emphases in the stories people tell. Of course "Some Get Mad" was itself my editorial suggestion, and the "original" manuscript I saw may already have been shaped in ways that modified Andersen's experience. The anecdote suggests both that there is little unedited experience available, but also that much anger is expressly edited out of illness stories.

27. Andersen writes that among friends and outsiders, Dick would return to his charming "old" self.

28. The idealization inherent in the communicative body is specified by M. Therese Lysaught, who applies my schema of body types in Sharing Christ's Passion: A Critique of the Role of Suffering in the Discourse of Bio-

medical Ethics from the Perspective of the Sick, Ph.D. diss., Duke University, 1992. Lysaught argues that the exemplar of the communicative body is Jesus, particularly in the crucifixion. This application of my work completely surprised me, and I gratefully acknowledge its importance in my present thinking.

29. Broyard, *Intoxicated by My Illness*, 45.

30. Schweitzer, *Out of My Life and Thought*, 104.

3. ILLNESS AS A CALL FOR STORIES

1. Roy Schafer, "Narration in the Psychoanalytic Dialogue," in W. J. T. Mitchell, ed., *On Narrative* (Chicago: University of Chicago Press, 1981), 31.

2. My title phrase comes from Coles, *The Call of Stories* (cf. chap. 2, n. 17). Coles's different emphasis describes how a moral life can be lived as the "call of stories," specifically literary stories that become woven into one's own life story.

3. Ronald Dworkin, *Life's Dominion: An Argument About Abortion, Euthanasia, and Individual Freedom* (New York: Knopf, 1993), 211. Dworkin refers specifically to the effects of prolonged immobility on the sense of self and the self's capacity for decision-making in matters such as termination of treatment.

4. Schafer, "Narration in Psychoanalytic Dialogue," 31.

5. Audre Lorde, *The Cancer Journals* (San Francisco: spinsters/*aunt lute*, 1980), 65.

6. In addition to sources cited below, see in particular George C. Rosenwald and Richard L. Ochberg, eds., *Storied Lives: The Cultural Politics of Self-Understanding* (New Haven: Yale University Press, 1992). A useful bibliography of recent work on narrative with reference to the self is found in Genevieve Lloyd, *Being in Time: Selves and Narrators in Philosophy and Literature* (New York: Routledge, 1993), 176.

7. The editors of the diaries of Etty Hillesum, a Dutch Jew who died in Auschwitz, captured this in their title, *An Interrupted Life* (New York: Washington Square Books, 1983). Recently, Susanna Kaysen calls her memoir of mental illness *Girl Interrupted* (New York: Vintage, 1993).

8. Nancy Mairs, *Ordinary Time: Cycles in Marriage, Faith, and Renewal* (Boston: Beacon Press, 1993), 122.

9. Roy Schafer, *Retelling a Life: Narration and Dialogue in Psychoanalysis* (New York: Basic Books, 1992), 32.

10. Richard Selzer, *Raising the Dead* (New York: Viking, 1992), 95.

11. Candice West, *Routine Complications: Troubles with Talk between Doctors and Patients* (Bloomington: Indiana University Press, 1984), and H. Beckman and R. Frankel, "The Effect of Physician Behavior on the Collection of Data," *Annals of Internal Medicine* 101 (1984): 692–96.

12. Howard Waitzkin, *The Politics of Medical Encounters: How Patients*

and Doctors Deal with Social Problems (New Haven: Yale University Press, 1991), 28.

13. Mairs, *Ordinary Time*, 100.

14. Fitzhugh Mullan, *Vital Signs: A Young Doctor's Struggle with Cancer* (New York: Laurel, 1984), 195.

15. Lloyd, *Being in Time*, 111.

16. David Carr, *Time, Narrative, and History* (Bloomington: Indiana University Press, 1986), 96.

17. Donald P. Spence, *Narrative Truth and Historical Truth: Meaning and Interpretation in Psychoanalysis* (New York: Norton, 1982), 31. See also Schafer: "Experience is made or fashioned; it is not encountered, discovered, or observed. . . . The introspecting subject extracts from the plenitude of potential experience what is wanted" (*Retelling a Life*, 23).

18. Roger C. Schank, *Tell Me a Story: A New Look at Real and Artificial Memory* (New York: Scribners, 1990), 115, original emphases changed.

19. Paul Ricoeur, "Life: A Story in Search of a Narrator," in M. C. Doeser and J. N. Kraay, eds., *Facts and Values* (Dordrecht: Martinus Nijhoff Publishers, 1986), 132.

20. Tim Brookes, *Catching My Breath: An Asthmatic Explores His Illness* (New York: Times Books, 1994), 277.

21. William F. May, *The Patient's Ordeal* (Bloomington: Indiana University Press, 1991), 131, see also 3.

22. Spence, *Narrative Truth and Historical Truth*, 31.

23. Lorde, *The Cancer Journals*, 22.

24. Kathryn Montgomery Hunter, *Doctors' Stories: The Narrative Structure of Medical Knowledge* (Princeton: Princeton University Press, 1991).

25. Lorde, *The Cancer Journals*, 65.

26. Jerome Bruner, *Acts of Meaning* (Cambridge: Harvard University Press, 1990), 109. Bruner is writing about Kenneth Gergen in this passage.

27. Waitzkin, *Politics of Medical Encounters*, 299–300, n. 8. Waitzkin is quoting Theron Britt.

28. Stewart Alsop, *Stay of Execution*, x (cf. chap. 2, n. 18).

29. Schafer, *Retelling a Life*, 26.

30. Sue Nathanson, *Soul Crisis: One Woman's Journey Through Abortion to Renewal* (New York: Signet, 1989), 209.

31. Schafer, *Retelling a Life*, 28.

32. Reynolds Price, *A Whole New Life* (New York: Atheneum, 1994), 183.

33. Lloyd, *Being in Time*, 20.

34. Anne Hunsaker Hawkins, in *Reconstructing Illness* (cf. chap. 1, n. 34), describes illness stories, or "pathographies," as the contemporary form of spiritual autobiographies, suggesting the former has displaced the latter. I see the spiritual autobiography as alive, well, and anything but displaced: Malcolm Boyd, Frederick Buechner, Annie Dillard, Richard Gilman,

Natalie Goldberg, Sam Keen, Madeleine L'Engle, Julius Lester, Kathleen Norris, and Dan Wakefield are only some of the many contemporary spiritual autobiographers. Illness stories and spiritual autobiographies seem rather to complement each other. Just as the illness story is a self-story reclaiming the post-colonial self's identity from medical systems, many spiritual autobiographies explore how to restore a spiritual impetus within religions that have ossified into formal systems. Illness and spiritual self-stories overlap in both Madeleine L'Engle, *Two-Part Invention: The Story of a Marriage* (New York: HarperCollins, 1989) and Nancy Mairs, *Ordinary Time*.

35. Self-stories of gender and of illness often weave together in AIDS narratives. In the work of Paul Monette, compare his story of gay identity, *Becoming a Man: Half a Life Story* (New York: HarperCollins, 1992), with *Borrowed Time: An AIDS Memoir* (New York: Avon, 1988) and *Last Watch of the Night* (New York: Harcourt Brace, 1994). Paul Zweig's *Departures: Memoirs* (New York: Penguin, 1986) is a gender story interrupted by illness, in his case lymphoma.

36. Incest-survivor stories probably do most to set the cultural threshold for personal writing; see Charlotte Vale Allen, *Daddy's Girl: A Very Personal Memoir* (New York: Bantam, 1981). Thus when Richard Selzer describes the writing in his illness memoir, *Raising the Dead*, as "so open, explicit, so personal" (29), he actually is far within the boundaries that survivor stories have set for open, explicit, and personal writing.

37. Clark Blaise, *I Had a Father: A Post-Modern Autobiography* (Toronto: HarperCollins, 1993), xi. Commenting on his usage of postmodern in his title, Blaise also notes that his reconstruction of his life cannot be linear.

38. Sam Keen, "Our Mythic Stories," in Charles and Anne Simpkinson, eds., *Sacred Stories: A Celebration of the Power of Stories to Transform and Heal* (New York: HarperCollins, 1993), 28. Note the postmodernity of the book's title: in an age of narrative wreckage, an enhanced belief in the efficacy of stories emerges.

39. Nancy Mairs, *Voice Lessons: On Becoming a (Woman) Writer* (Boston: Beacon Press, 1994), 15.

40. Terry Tempest Williams, *Refuge: An Unnatural History of Family and Place* (New York: Vintage, 1991).

41. See Gareth Williams, "The Genesis of Chronic Illness: Narrative Reconstruction," *Sociology of Health and Illness* 6, no. 2 (1984): 175–200.

42. On the need for a postmodern social science as a means of grasping the distortions of language that—however presciently observed by George Orwell—took on a new quantity and intensity during the Vietnam war era, see Charles Lemert, "The Uses of French Structuralism in Sociology," in George Ritzer, ed., *Frontiers of Social Theory: The New Synthesis* (New York: Columbia University Press, 1990), 230–54.

4. THE RESTITUTION NARRATIVE

1. Friedrich Nietzsche, *The Gay Science*, trans. Walter Kaufmann (New York: Vintage, 1974), 249–50. This passage is discussed in detail in chapter 6, section 1.

2. One other type could be called the political/environmental narrative. Here the ill person presents herself as having been made ill by toxins originating usually in some specific industry. Bill's narrative in Williams, "The Genesis of Chronic Illness" (cf. chap. 3, n. 41), would fit this type, as would the stories reported by Balshem, *Cancer in the Community* (cf. chap. 1, n. 20). Investigative reporting on pollution often contains such narratives; see Monte Paulsen, "The Politics of Cancer: Why the Medical Establishment Blames Victims instead of Carcinogens," *Utne Reader,* November/ December 1993, 81–89. Susan DiGiacomo proposes one variant of this form, the "victimization narrative." Here identity derives from being a victim of some person, group, or institution, and the narrative telos involves punishing that victimizer (personal communication). Another variant is what Anne Hunsaker Hawkins calls the "ecological narrative" in which the genesis of illness progressively expands in a web of connections that is both extensive and dense (personal communication).

3. May, *The Patient's Ordeal,* 4 (cf. chap. 3, n. 21).

4. Talcott Parsons, *The Social System* (New York: Free Press, 1951). The sick role receives its last and fullest elaboration in *Action Theory and the Human Condition* (New York: Free Press: 1978), chapters 1–3. For the aspects of Parsons's theory that move into postmodernity, see my article, "From Sick Role to Health Role: Deconstructing Parsons," in R. Robertson and B. S. Turner, eds., *Talcott Parsons: Theorist of Modernity* (London: Sage, 1991), 205–16.

5. Late in his life Parsons became diabetic. He suggests this experience did not modify his earlier theory substantially. See *Action Theory,* 19, 20, 25, 27, 29.

6. Or, more curious to the layman, the specialists might agree that treatment was futile but still believe they had to do *something.* For sociological reports on such attitudes, see Charles Bosk, *All God's Mistakes: Genetic Counseling in a Pediatric Hospital* (Chicago: University of Chicago Press, 1992) and Zussman, *Intensive Care* (cf. chap. 2, n. 9). One physician's struggle with his colleagues' obsession to continue treating is told in Harold Klawans, *Life, Death, and In Between* (New York: Paragon House, 1992), 259–70. For a medical ethicist writing on pressures to continue treatment of comatose patients exerted by their families who are caught in a restitution narrative, see Nancy Dubler and David Nimmons, *Ethics on Call* (New York: Harmony Books, 1992), 32–33, 334–37.

7. For a similar story, see Sherwin B. Nuland, *How We Die: Reflections on Life's Final Chapter* (New York: Knopf, 1994), 250–54.

8. Bauman, *Mortality, Immortality and Other Life Strategies* (cf. chap. 1, n. 25). Bauman's critique of modernist medicine stands almost alone in its post-Parsonian stance; to achieve this stance Bauman had to situate his critique of medicine within a more general critique of modernity. For a different postmodernist perspective, see Nicholas Fox, *Postmodernism, Sociology, and Health* (Toronto: University of Toronto Press, 1994).

9. Nuland calls medical puzzles The Riddle: "The Riddle is the doctor's lodestone as an applied scientist; it is his albatross as a humane caregiver" (*How We Die*, 260).

10. Nicholas Regush, *Safety Last: The Failure of the Consumer Health Protection System in Canada* (Toronto: Key Porter, 1993).

11. Mark Lowry, "Cancer Warrior," *Calgary Herald*, April 30, 1994. The story is a variant of Regush's "gee whiz" genre, although the commodity is expertise as individual genius, not some technological product.

12. Quoted in Bauman, *Mortality, Immortality*, 162.

13. Sharon Adams, "Sick Over Silicon," *Calgary Herald*, April 30, 1994.

14. The stories alternate between DiGiacomo's victimization stories and what I will call, in the next chapter, chaos stories.

15. Schweitzer, *Out of My Life and Thought*, 195 (cf. chap. 2, n. 11).

16. Zussman, *Intensive Care*, 61.

17. Ibid., 60. Parsons was explicit about this "primary importance" from the patient's side; he refers to "a definite responsibility on the patient in working toward the common goals of the system as a whole" (*Action Theory*, 25).

18. Bauman, *Mortality, Immortality*, 209.

19. This "postmodern" attitude is as old as the moral dilemma of Sophocles' *Antigone*. One example of the voice of the "moral person" as it is heard in professional medicine is the Israeli physician and medical educator Shimon Glick, who writes, in terms that echo Bauman, "Basically, the modern world in which we live has set for itself an order of priorities that does not demand meticulous examination of behavior by a rigorous, ethical standard" ("The Empathic Physician," in Spiro, *Empathy and the Practice of Medicine*, 100 [cf. Preface, n. 3]).

20. Nuland, *How We Die*, 244. In this passage Nuland reflects not on the deaths of his patients, but on how he and his family managed the death of his beloved grandmother. For my own story of my mother-in-law's death, see "Interrupted Stories, Interrupted Lives," *Second Opinion* 20 (July 1994): 11–18.

21. For arguments developing this contradiction, see William Gaylin, "Faulty Diagnosis: Why Clinton's Health-Care Plan Won't Cure What Ails Us," *Harper's*, October 1993, 57–64. On the incapacity of the individualist model of "traditional medicine" to address the health issues of the poorest members of society, see Hilfiker, *Not All of Us Are Saints*, 151, 176, 211 (cf. chap. 2, n. 21).

22. Bauman, *Mortality, Immortality,* 129–30, emphases added.

23. Other influential physicians calling for change in medical moral orientations include Howard Brody, *The Healer's Power* (New Haven: Yale University Press, 1992); Eric Cassell, *The Nature of Suffering and the Goals of Medicine* (New York: Oxford University Press, 1991); Ron Charach, ed., *The Naked Physician: Poems About the Lives of Patients and Doctors* (Kingston, Ontario and Clayton, New York: Quarry Press, 1990); Coles, *The Call of Stories* (cf. chap. 2, n. 17); Kleinman, *The Illness Narratives* (cf. Preface, n. 2); Spiro, *Empathy and the Practice of Medicine;* and Waitzkin, *The Politics of Medical Encounters* (cf. chap. 3, n. 12).

5. THE CHAOS NARRATIVE

1. I am especially in debt to Lawrence L. Langer, *Holocaust Testimonies: the Ruins of Memory* (cf. Epigraph, n. 1).

2. Kathy Charmaz, *Good Days, Bad Days: The Self in Chronic Illness and Time* (Berkeley: University of California Press, 1991), 173.

3. Radner, *It's Always Something,* 112 (cf. chap. 2, n. 10).

4. Barb Livingston, "Legacy of Anger Lingers On," *Herald Sunday Magazine,* May 26, 1991, 10. My meetings with support groups devoted to endometriosis and chronic fatigue syndrome underscored for me the general mistrust that people with such diseases have of medicine. Yet the same people also hang on news of treatment "breakthroughs."

5. Langer, *Holocaust Testimonies,* 35, see also 2; for an example of such steering by the interviewer, see 58–60.

6. Primo Levi, *The Drowned and the Saved,* trans. Raymond Rosenthal (New York: Vintage, 1988), 157.

7. David Hilfiker analyzes the frustration he feels with his destitute patients' inability to do what medicine presupposes patients ought to do, help themselves. Helping themselves, Hilfiker realizes, is exactly what their condition of destitution has rendered them incapable of. See his *Not All of Us Are Saints,* especially chapter 7, "Victims of Victims" (cf. chap. 2, n. 21).

8. Elaine Scarry, *The Body in Pain: The Making and Unmaking of the World* (New York: Oxford University Press, 1985). I return to Scarry in chapter 8.

9. Flaubert's story "The Legend of St. Julian Hospitator" is perhaps the finest literary evocation of such a gesture, when Julian finally overcomes his abhorrence and embraces the Leper, thus winning a vision of Christ. Gustave Flaubert, *Three Tales,* trans. Robert Baldick (New York: Penguin, 1961), 57–87. For a contemporary account of trying to live according to this ideal, see David Hilfiker, whose title, *Not All of Us Are Saints,* suggests the conflicts and dilemmas of being a communicative body.

10. Langer, *Holocaust Testimonies,* 67.

11. For discussion of Sacks's accident, see chapter 6.

12. Oliver Sacks, *A Leg to Stand On* (New York: Summit Books, 1984), 126, 143–44.

13. In Kahane, *No Less a Woman* (cf. chap. 2, n. 23), these feelings are reported by Sarah (28) and Valerie (41).

14. While the interviewees described in Williams, "The Genesis of Chronic Illness," have elements of chaos in their stories, their sense of genesis orders their experience and thus is part of what keeps the chaos from dominating. On the indeterminacy of genesis, see Byron J. Good, "A Body in Chronic Pain—The Making of a World of Chronic Pain," in Mary-Jo DelVecchio Good et al., eds., *Pain as Human Experience: An Anthropological Perspective* (Berkeley: University of California Press, 1992), 29–48. Insofar as the father and son Good describe do patch together a story that gives the son's illness a genesis, that storytelling preserves them from the chaos that chronic pain could bring.

15. My paper "The Pedagogy of Suffering" (cf. chap. 1, n. 38) considers how psychooncology practices clinical reframings of patients' chaos stories.

16. Robert Bly, *Iron John: A Book About Men* (Reading, Mass.: Addison Wesley, 1990), 80.

17. Hilfiker, *Not All of Us Are Saints,* 210.

18. The same point is made by Waitzkin in his study of how medical interview talk steers patients toward some stories and away from others. Waitzkin concludes by considering non-North American medical systems where personal health is considered tied to social conditions. See his *Politics of Medical Encounters,* part 3, "Medical Micropolitics and Social Change," 257–77 (cf. chap. 3, n. 12).

19. Hilfiker, *Not All of Us Are Saints,* 212.

20. Frederick Franck, *A Little Compendium On That Which Matters* (New York: St. Martin's Press, 1993), 14.

6. The Quest Narrative

1. John Donne, *Devotions upon Emergent Occasions* (1624; Ann Arbor: University of Michigan Press, 1959).

2. Nietzsche, *The Gay Science,* 249–50 (cf. chap. 4, n. 1).

3. David B. Morris, *The Culture of Pain* (Berkeley: University of California Press, 1991), 284. Morris goes on to write of "defiance" as "among the most important stances that may come to characterize the new postmodern attitudes toward pain" (285).

4. Broyard, *Intoxicated by My Illness,* 47–48, see also 29 (cf. chap. 2, n. 20).

5. Joseph Campbell, *The Hero With a Thousand Faces* (1949; Princeton: Princeton University Press, 1972).

6. Hawkins recognizes Campbell as a central influence on the stories she discusses in her chapter, "Myths of Battle and Journey," *Reconstructing Ill-*

ness, 61–90 (cf. chap. 1, n. 34). She situates Campbell in an anthropological tradition of scholars concerned with initiation and rites of passage (85). The influence I attribute to *Hero With a Thousand Faces* has little to do with whether Campbell is reporting myths or creating one.

7. As Campbell neatly phrases the hero's identity, "it is found (or rather, recollected) that the hero himself is that which he had come to find" (*Hero With a Thousand Faces*, 163).

8. Nathanson, *Soul Crisis*, 282 (cf. chap. 3, n. 30). The initiation metaphor is also used explicitly in Kat Duff, *The Alchemy of Illness* (New York: Pantheon, 1993). Duff describes the stages of initiation as being "separation, submergence, metamorphosis, and reemergence" (93), following Campbell, who is her primary citation.

9. Linda Garro, "Chronic Illness and the Construction of Narratives," in Good et al., eds., *Pain as Human Experience*, 129 (cf. chap. 5, n. 14).

10. Again, the reasons why Campbell seems to work are overdetermined: tellers may have read the myths that inform Campbell's work, or they may have read Campbell, or Campbell may be such a part of contemporary narrative common capital that his influence is just there, or, alternatively, there may be an archetypal structure to experience.

11. See Hawkins's bibliography, *Reconstructing Illness*, 166–67 (cf. chap. 1, n. 34), for an array of "conquering" titles, including: *How I Conquered Cancer Naturally, I Beat Cancer,* and *The Cancer Conqueror: An Incredible Journey to Wellness.* Some of these titles and subtitles reflect the marketing strategies of editors and publicists; others reflect the storyteller's self-perception as an ill person, or as a distinctly *former* ill person. Still other titles may be more subtle. When Max Lerner subtitled his book *A Memoir of My Triumph Over Illness*, the triumph seems more spiritual than physical. See his *Wrestling With the Angel* (New York: Norton, 1990). The importance of all these titles, however they are intended, is that they create the culture of illness that other ill people have to negotiate as this culture is enacted in expectations of self and others.

12. Campbell writes, "We are all reflexes of the image of the Bodhisattva. The sufferer within us is that divine being. We and the protecting father are one. This is the redeeming insight. That protecting father is every man we meet" (*Hero With a Thousand Faces*, 161). With respect to the masculine language of this passage, note that the Bodhisattva is explicitly androgynous (152). See also James D. Thomas, "The Bodhisattva as Metaphor to Jung's Concept of Self" in David J. Meckel and Robert L. Moore, eds. *Self and Liberation: The Jung-Buddhist Dialogue* (New York: Paulist Press, 1992), 206–31.

13. Campbell, *Hero With a Thousand Faces*, 147, 162, 260.

14. Ibid., 308. This line could be the opening for a strong critique of many of the New Age appropriations of the "journey" narrative.

15. William Styron, *Darkness Visible: A Memoir of Madness* (New York: Random House, 1990). Styron's "coming out" subtitle carries more than a hint of provocation.

16. John Updike, "At War with My Skin," in *Self-Consciousness: Memoirs* (New York: Fawcett Crest, 1989), 42–80.

17. Radner, *It's Always Something,* 145 (cf. chap. 2, n. 10).

18. Audre Lorde, *The Cancer Journals,* 59 (cf. chap. 3, n. 5).

19. Irving Zola, *Missing Pieces: A Chronicle of Living With a Disability* (Philadelphia: Temple University Press, 1982).

20. Another example of a disability story in the prophetic voice is Barbara Webster, *All of a Piece: A Life with Multiple Sclerosis* (Baltimore: Johns Hopkins University Press, 1989).

21. I take this term from Paul Zweig, *Three Journeys: An Automythology* (New York: Basic Books, 1976).

22. William May, *The Patient's Ordeal,* 22 (cf. chap. 3, n. 21).

23. Sacks, *A Leg to Stand On,* 197 (cf. chap. 5, n. 12).

24. Norman Cousins, *Anatomy of an Illness as Perceived by the Patient: Reflections on Healing and Regeneration* (New York: Bantam, 1981). Cousins later suffered a heart attack which he wrote about in *The Healing Heart* (New York: Avon, 1983). The latter book draws on the automythology of the former one, and the story of the initial cardiac incident depends on everyone involved recognizing the patient as *the* Norman Cousins. Cousins acknowledges his particular status but never fully engages its significance in his treatment. Heroes rarely acknowledge all that makes themselves possible, those qualities being what the rest of us are left to puzzle out and seek to emulate.

25. Lorde, *The Cancer Journals,* 61.

26. L'Engle, *Two-Part Invention,* 229, 181 (cf. chap. 3, n. 34).

27. Kahane, *No Less a Woman,* 83 (cf. chap. 2, n. 23).

28. Sacks, *A Leg to Stand On,* 219.

29. My initial usage of this phrase occurs in "The Rhetoric of Self-Change: Illness Experience as Narrative," *The Sociological Quarterly* 34, no. 1 (1993): 39–52.

30. Lorde, *The Cancer Journals,* 35; see also 45.

31. Robert F. Murphy, *The Body Silent* (New York: Henry Holt, 1987), ix.

32. Lorde, *The Cancer Journals,* 59.

33. Ibid., 20.

34. See the discussion above of Zussman, *Intensive Care* (cf. chap. 2, n. 9). Although Zussman continues to privilege the physician as modernist hero, he also recognizes the real costs of this heroism.

35. See chapter 4, above; Bauman, *Mortality, Immortality,* 209 (cf. chap. 1, n. 25).

36. Paul Ricoeur, *Essays on Biblical Interpretation* (Philadelphia: Fortress Press, 1980), 131.

37. May, *The Patient's Ordeal,* 24.

38. Langer, *Holocaust Memories,* 3 (cf. Epigraph, n. 1).

7. TESTIMONY

1. One among many critiques of frustrated testimony refers to "dysfunctional narratives." See Charles Baxter, "No-Fault Fiction: Blame the Presidents," *Harper's,* November 1994, 13–15. In these narratives responsibility is absent; evil is named but never judged: "What we have instead is not exactly drama and not exactly therapy. It exists between the two, very much of our time, where deniability reigns" (14). This book is not about dysfunctional narratives, but the testimonies I do describe are made more necessary against this background. It is melodramatic but perhaps not wrong to suggest that the soul of postmodern times is contested between forms of testimony: those that tell suppressed truths and those that in seeming to tell such truths actually perpetuate denial; not just specific denials to particular evils, but a culture of denial. Among illness stories, the prevalent form of "dysfunctional narratives" are restitution stories that continue to be told after hope of restitution has passed, thus negating the responsibilities of the dying and those around her; see chapter 4.

2. Shoshana Felman, "Education and Crisis," in Felman and Dori Laub, *Testimony: Crises of Witnessing in Literature, Psychoanalysis, and History* (New York: Routledge, 1992), 5. Felman and Laub attempt no canonical definition of testimony, and I follow their wise example. Testimony is best left in its particulars; its various forms are "like snowflakes," in Susan DiGiacomo's elegant phrase (personal communication).

3. Art Spiegelman, *Maus: A Survivor's Tale. I. My Father Bleeds History* and *II. And Here My Troubles Began* (New York: Pantheon, 1986 and 1991).

4. Jean-François Lyotard, *The Postmodern Condition,* trans. Geoff Bennington and Brian Massumi (Minneapolis: University of Minnesota Press, 1984).

5. Gabriel Marcel, *The Mystery of Being,* vol. 2, *Faith and Reality,* trans. Rene Hague (Chicago: Henry Regnery, 1960), 144. My appreciation to Jamie S. Scott for pointing out these quotations.

6. Garro, "Chronic Illness and the Construction of Narratives," 129 (cf. chap. 6, n. 9).

7. Jodi Halpern, "Empathy: Using Resonance Emotions in the Service of Curiosity," in Spiro et al., *Empathy and the Practice of Medicine,* 169 (cf. Preface, n. 3).

8. Although deconstruction is practiced most famously by Jacques Derrida, the tendency I refer to here has its source in Roland Barthes, "The Death of the Author," *Image-Music-Text,* trans. Stephen Heath (New York: Hill & Wang, 1983), 142–48.

9. See Dorothy Smith, *The Conceptual Practices of Power* (Toronto: Uni-

versity of Toronto Press, 1990). Smith's theories are applied to medical settings by Timothy Diamond, *Making Gray Gold: Narratives of Nursing Home Care* (Chicago: University of Chicago Press, 1992).

10. Halpern, quoted above, is a physician. On the physician as witness, see in particular Rita Charon, "To Listen, To Recognize," *The Pharos of Alpha Omega Alpha* 49, no. 4 (Fall 1986): 10–13. Charon refers back to the physician portrayed in John Berger's *A Fortunate Man,* who describes himself as "clerk" of his patients' records, which are their life records, not just their medical charts. Arthur Kleinman has written extensively on the physician as witness; see *The Illness Narratives,* 168–69 (cf. Preface, n. 2), for a moving doctor's story of the need to witness and what impedes witnessing in professional work.

11. Calls by physicians for a new conceptualization of suffering include Kleinman, *The Illness Narratives;* Eric J. Cassell, *The Nature of Suffering and the Goals of Medicine* (cf. chap. 4, n. 23); and, from a different perspective, Timothy E. Quill, *Death and Dignity: Making Choices and Taking Charge* (New York: W. W. Norton, 1993). Note that these voices remain controversial. I attended a conference where Cassell spoke; at the closing plenary session another physician ridiculed his emphasis on suffering, saying that he himself "preferred joy." Although the conference concerned doctor/patient communication, no ill people were invited to speak.

12. Donald N. Levine, *The Flight from Ambiguity* (Chicago: University of Chicago Press, 1985).

13. Jürgen Habermas, *The Theory of Communicative Action,* vol. 2, *Lifeworld and System,* trans. Thomas McCarthy (Boston: Beacon Press, 1987).

14. Bosk, *All God's Mistakes,* 171 (cf. chap. 4, n. 6).

15. Zussman, *Intensive Care,* 43 (cf. chap. 2, n. 9).

16. Others tell a different story. David Hilfiker not only provides numerous anecdotes of his medical colleagues' prejudices and how these affected treatment, but he also describes with extraordinary honesty his own difficulty in trying to rid himself of biases against those whom he perceives as responsible, even in part, for their own illness. See Hilfiker, *Not All of Us Are Saints,* especially 99–103, 162–63 (cf. chap. 2, n. 21). For accounts of medical moralizing in the care of AIDS, see Abraham Verghese, *My Own Country: A Doctor's Story of a Town and its People in the Age of AIDS* (New York: Simon and Schuster, 1994), 88, 131, 183, 206–7.

17. For one story of this activism, see Sharon Batt, *Patient No More: The Politics of Breast Cancer* (Charlottetown, P.E.I.: Ragweed Press, 1994).

18. Mairs, *Ordinary Time,* 163 (cf. chap. 3, n. 8).

19. Hilfiker, *Not All of Us Are Saints,* 188. See also Jean Vanier, *The Broken Body: Journey to Wholeness* (New York: Paulist Press, 1988). Vanier is founder of L'Arche communities for people with mental disabilities.

20. Edith Stein, a philosopher, writes, "A 'we,' not an 'I,' is the subject of

the empathizing." Quoted in Helle Mathiasen and Joseph S. Alpert, "Lessons in Empathy: Literature, Art, and Medicine" in Spiro et al., *Empathy and the Practice of Medicine,* 140. Stein's observation reflects earlier writings of Martin Buber, and Max Scheler, among others.

21. Joan Tronto, *Moral Boundaries: A Political Argument for an Ethic of Care* (New York: Routledge, 1993), 7.

22. Diamond, *Making Gray Gold,* 162.

23. György Lukács, *Soul and Form,* trans. Anna Bostok (London: Merlin Press, 1974), 57. Also quoted by Bauman, *Mortality, Immortality,* 203 (cf. chap. 1, n. 25).

24. Hilfiker, *Not All of Us Are Saints,* 188.

25. Rita Charon, "Narrative Contributions to Medical Ethics: Recognition, Formulation, Interpretation, and Validation in the Practice of the Ethicist" in Edwin R. DuBose, Ron Hamel, and Laurence J. O'Connell, eds., *A Matter of Principles: Ferment in U.S. Bioethics* (Valley Forge: Trinity International Press, 1994), 277.

26. For a complementary argument on the contributions of a grounding in narrative for medical practice, see Helle Mathiasen and Joseph S. Alpert, "Lessons in Empathy: Literature, Art, and Medicine," in Spiro et al., *Empathy and the Practice of Medicine,* 135–59.

27. Kleinman, *The Illness Narratives,* 39. For another example of a physician called to a personal relationship with someone who, in that relationship, ceased to be his patient, see 146–49.

28. Charon is equally aware of the moral commitment inherent in the physician's calling; thus she specifies that "every physician-patient encounter involves a moral dimension" (264). See also "To Listen, To Recognize."

29. See Kathryn Montgomery Hunter and Steven H. Miles, "Commentary," and Miles, "Overview," *Second Opinion* 15 (November 1990): 60–67. These articles introduced Hunter and Miles's editorship of the "Case Stories" series, 1990–93.

30. Barry Hoffmaster, "The Forms and Limits of Medical Ethics," *Social Science and Medicine* 39, no. 9 (1994): 1161.

31. See Blaise, *I Had a Father* (cf. chap. 3, n. 37), for one postmodern tale of the impossibility of sorting out good and bad, virtuous and non-virtuous; in this instance the question is the moral identity of Blaise's father and how this identity affects Blaise's own moral self.

32. For a history of how medical textbooks have instructed doctors to treat patient stories, see David Armstrong, "The Patient's View," *Social Science and Medicine* 18 (1984): 737–44. The clinical medical view was complemented, in the 1950s, by a social scientific appropriation of the patient's story. Armstrong concludes, "the patient's view is an artifact of socio-medical perception." For a detailed analysis of the examining-room talk in which patient stories are transformed into medical records, see Waitzkin, *The Politics*

of Medical Encounters (cf. chap. 3, n. 12). For analysis of medical case presentations and how these replace the agency of the ill person with that of medical technology, relegating the patient to the passive voice, see Renée Anspach, "Notes on the Sociology of Medical Discourse: The Language of Case Presentation," *Journal of Health and Social Behavior* 29 (December 1988): 357–75.

33. Halpern, "Empathy: Using Resonance Emotions in the Service of Curiosity."

34. Martha Nussbaum, "Narrative Emotions: Beckett's Genealogy of Love," in Stanley Hauerwas and L. Gregory Jones, eds., *Why Narrative? Readings in Narrative Theology* (Grand Rapids, Michigan: Eerdmans, 1989), 247–48.

35. Steven H. Miles, "The Case: A Story Lost and Found," *Second Opinion* 15 (November 1990): 55–59. An especially sensitive discussion of the end-of-life as a culmination of what the life has meant is found in Dworkin, *Life's Dominion,* especially 199–217 (cf. chap. 3, n. 3).

36. Alsop, *Stay of Execution,* 259, 288 (cf. chap. 2, n. 18).

37. Ibid., 290; for an earlier story of someone dying at sixty, see 210.

38. In social scientific terms, the difference is between the research proposal that requires the results be indicated in advance versus research that seeks to discover the parameters of investigation in the course of investigating. This difference is no longer simply quantitative versus qualitative; thus I think of it as modernist versus postmodern. Modernity thinks it knows the parameters in advance and only needs data to support anticipated conclusions. Postmodernity tends to regard finding the parameters *as* the conclusion, and accepts that its own investigations have created these parameters through the investigating.

39. Here I take a slightly different line than Bauman, *Mortality, Immortality,* 162–64, although Bauman's discussion of projects instigates my comments.

40. Frederick Franck, *A Little Compendium On That Which Matters,* 7 (cf. chap. 5, n. 20).

41. Mairs, *Ordinary Time,* 217 .

42. Lorde, *The Cancer Journals,* 20 (cf. chap. 3, n. 5).

8. THE WOUND AS HALF OPENING

1. Cassell, *The Nature of Suffering and the Goals of Medicine,* 33 (cf. chap. 4, n. 23).

2. Arthur Kleinman, "Pain and Resistance: The Delegitimation and Relegitimation of Local Worlds," in Good et. al., eds., *Pain as Human Experience,* 174 (cf. chap. 5, n. 14).

3. Arthur W. Frank, "Cyberpunk Bodies and Postmodern Times," *Studies in Symbolic Interaction* 13 (1992): 39–50.

4. Providers confirm the legitimacy of this paranoia; see Dubler and Nimmons, *Ethics On Call* (cf. chap. 4, n. 6)

5. Scarry, *The Body in Pain* (cf. chap. 5, n. 8). In particular my discussions with Susan DiGiacomo have shaped my thoughts about torture. I consider the analogy in an earlier article, "The Rhetoric of Self-Change: Illness Experience as Narrative" (cf. chap. 6, n. 29).

6. Kahane, *No Less a Woman,* 122 (cf. chap. 2, n. 23).

7. Scarry, *The Body in Pain,* 47.

8. Zussman, *Intensive Care,* 109–15 (cf. chap. 2, n. 9).

9. Ibid., 111; Perri Klass, *A Not Entirely Benign Procedure* (New York: Signet, 1988), 240–41; Quill, *Death and Dignity,* 57–58 (cf. chap. 7, n. 11).

10. At the end of support group meetings when all sorts of resentments against medicine have been expressed, organizers have told me that their largest attendance turns out to hear physicians who might promise some new treatment.

11. Lerner, *Wrestling With the Angel,* 56 (cf. chap. 6, n. 11).

12. Ricoeur, "Life: A Story in Search of a Narrator," 131 (cf. chap. 3, n. 19).

13. Emmanuel Levinas, "Useless Suffering," trans. Richard A. Cohen, *The Provocation of Levinas: Rethinking the Other,* ed. Robert Bernasconi and David Wood (London: Routledge: 1988), 158.

14. For a summary of the Jacob story that raises this issue, see Reynolds Price, "A Single Meaning: Notes on the Origins and Life of Narrative," *A Common Room: Essays 1954–1987* (New York: Atheneum, 1989), 259–62. For my earlier invocation of the Jacob story, see *At the Will of the Body,* 80–82 (cf. chap. 1, n. 12).

15. Levinas, "Useless Suffering," 163.

16. The "category of the medical" is also explicated by Levinas when he refers in the long quotation above to the "original call for aid, for curative help" being directed to "the other ego whose alterity, whose exteriority promises salvation." Thus Levinas supports, at least as an abstract principle, William Osler's often-repeated advice to young physicians of 1932 that they practice "imperturbability" (quoted and discussed in Richard L. Landau, " . . . And the Least of These is Empathy," in Spiro et al., *Empathy and the Practice of Medicine,* 103–9 [cf. Preface, n. 3]). The problem of practice is whether contemporary medicine retains the ethical context that Levinas presupposes of being *for* the other. The one, perhaps a physician, whose exteriority is to the sufferer a promise of salvation must also define herself as existing *for* that sufferer, an attitude described above (chap. 7, "The Pedagogy of Suffering") as the physician as servant. Imperturbability may be the grace of a servant, but it is also the insufferable arrogance of a master.

17. Garro, "Chronic Illness and the Construction of Narratives," 129 (cf. chap. 5, n. 14).

18. Quoted by Michael Lerner, *Choices in Healing: Integrating the Best of*

Conventional and Complementary Approaches to Cancer (Cambridge: MIT Press, 1994), 124. A parallel statement is found in Rachel Naomi Remen, *On Healing* (Bolinas, Calif.: The Institute for the Study of Health and Illness, 1993), no page numbers.

19. Dennis Kaye, *Laugh, I Thought I'd Die: My Life with ALS.* (Toronto: Viking, 1993), 260. Also personal communication, for which I am profoundly grateful.

Index

145 note pedagogs & suffering used differently
mine eyes ...